CANCER ETIOLOGY, DIAGNOSIS AND TREATMENTS

A BIOCHEMICAL VIEW OF HEAD AND NECK CANCERS

CANCER ETIOLOGY, DIAGNOSIS AND TREATMENTS

Additional books and e-books in this series can be found on Nova's website under the Series tab.

CANCER ETIOLOGY, DIAGNOSIS AND TREATMENTS

A BIOCHEMICAL VIEW OF HEAD AND NECK CANCERS

DOROTA BARTUSIK-AEBISHER
AND
DAVID AEBISHER
EDITORS

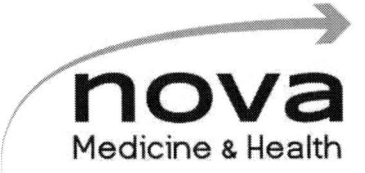

Copyright © 2021 by Nova Science Publishers, Inc.

All rights reserved. No part of this book may be reproduced, stored in a retrieval system or transmitted in any form or by any means: electronic, electrostatic, magnetic, tape, mechanical photocopying, recording or otherwise without the written permission of the Publisher.

We have partnered with Copyright Clearance Center to make it easy for you to obtain permissions to reuse content from this publication. Simply navigate to this publication's page on Nova's website and locate the "Get Permission" button below the title description. This button is linked directly to the title's permission page on copyright.com. Alternatively, you can visit copyright.com and search by title, ISBN, or ISSN.

For further questions about using the service on copyright.com, please contact:
Copyright Clearance Center
Phone: +1-(978) 750-8400　　　Fax: +1-(978) 750-4470　　　E-mail: info@copyright.com.

NOTICE TO THE READER

The Publisher has taken reasonable care in the preparation of this book, but makes no expressed or implied warranty of any kind and assumes no responsibility for any errors or omissions. No liability is assumed for incidental or consequential damages in connection with or arising out of information contained in this book. The Publisher shall not be liable for any special, consequential, or exemplary damages resulting, in whole or in part, from the readers' use of, or reliance upon, this material. Any parts of this book based on government reports are so indicated and copyright is claimed for those parts to the extent applicable to compilations of such works.

Independent verification should be sought for any data, advice or recommendations contained in this book. In addition, no responsibility is assumed by the Publisher for any injury and/or damage to persons or property arising from any methods, products, instructions, ideas or otherwise contained in this publication.

This publication is designed to provide accurate and authoritative information with regard to the subject matter covered herein. It is sold with the clear understanding that the Publisher is not engaged in rendering legal or any other professional services. If legal or any other expert assistance is required, the services of a competent person should be sought. FROM A DECLARATION OF PARTICIPANTS JOINTLY ADOPTED BY A COMMITTEE OF THE AMERICAN BAR ASSOCIATION AND A COMMITTEE OF PUBLISHERS.

Additional color graphics may be available in the e-book version of this book.

Library of Congress Cataloging-in-Publication Data

ISBN: 978-1-53619-370-1

Published by Nova Science Publishers, Inc. † New York

Contents

Preface		vii
Chapter 1	Biochemical Studies of Head Cancers *Lidia Bieniasz, David Aebisher, Wojciech Domka and Dorota Bartusik-Aebisher*	1
Chapter 2	Biochemical Studies of Neck Cancers *Lidia Bieniasz, David Aebisher, Wojciech Domka and Dorota Bartusik-Aebisher*	27
Chapter 3	Biochemical Studies of Head and Neck Cancer Treatments *Lidia Bieniasz, David Aebisher, Wojciech Domka and Dorota Bartusik-Aebisher*	51
Chapter 4	Biochemical Studies of Head and Neck Cancer Biomarkers *Wojciech Domka, David Aebisher, Lidia Bieniasz and Dorota Bartusik-Aebisher*	69
Chapter 5	Photomedicine of Head and Neck Cancer *Wojciech Domka, David Aebisher, Lidia Bieniasz and Dorota Bartusik-Aebisher*	81

Chapter 6	The Use of Laser Light in Laryngology *Wojciech Domka, David Aebisher, Lidia Bieniasz* *and Dorota Bartusik-Aebisher*	**113**
About the Editors		**139**
Index		**141**

PREFACE

This book addresses major problem in the management of patients with cancer of the head and neck. The authors have written six chapters of particular importance for head and neck cancer diagnosis, treatment, and rehabilitation. Chapter 1 describes treatment of patients with squamous cell carcinoma of the head. Chapter 2 presents treatment of patients with squamous cell carcinoma of the neck. Biochemical studies of head and neck cancer treatments are presented in Chaper 3. In chapter 4 biochemical studies of head and neck cancer biomarkers are presented. Photodynamic therapy (PDT) exploits light interactions and photosensitizers to induce cytotoxic reactive oxygen species. Photodynamic diagnosis (PDD) uses the phenomenon of photosensitizer emitting fluorescence to distinguish some tumors from normal tissue. PDT offers a therapeutic solution that has been found to be cost-effective compared to palliative major surgery or chemotherapy. However, despite the significant improvement noted in preclinical and clinical trials, PDT is still not considered the standard treatment option for head and neck cancer. Multiple photosensitizers have been studied and tumors have been treated in a variety of head and neck sites over the last 30 years. Photodynamic therapy is a palliative treatment option for head and neck squamous cell carcinoma patients which induces local inflammation and alters tumor cell morphology.

Chapter 1 - Treatment of patients with squamous cell carcinoma of the head is a significant problem. Head cancers are among the most common cancers. Every year, more than half a million cases of squamous cell carcinoma of the head and neck are reported worldwide, mainly involving the mouth and throat, lower pharynx and larynx.

Chapter 2 - Neck cancer is common in several regions of the World. However, most neck cancers occur in people older than 45. Neck cancer is relatively rare in women under the age of 45. Neck cancer risk is reduced by quitting smoking, and by reducing exposure to carcinogens in the environment. The most common symptom of neck cancer was difficulty breathing and stridor, followed by voice alteration and dysphagia.

Chapter 3 - Head and neck squamous cell carcinoma is an aggressive malignancy with high morbidity and mortality. Initial cancer assessment includes assessment of the histological appearance, tumor grading, lymph nodes status, and the presence of metastases. However, traditional diagnostic methods such as histopathology and radiology are not sensitive enough to detect a small number of neoplastic cells and are limited in their ability to predict treatment response. Recently, there has been significant progress in molecular diagnostics in these areas.

Chapter 4 - Cancer cells represent a specific metabolic state. Targeted therapies are urgently needed in order to minimize the treatment toxicity.

Chapter 5 - Photodynamic therapy (PDT) exploits light interactions and photosensitizers to induce cytotoxic reactive oxygen species. Photodynamic diagnosis (PDD) uses the phenomenon of photosensitizer emitting fluorescence to distinguish some tumors from normal tissue. The standard photosensitizer used for PDD is 5-aminolevulinic acid, although it is not entirely satisfactory. Many other targeted therapy strategies and medications are currently under investigation.

Chapter 6 - Photodynamic therapy (PDT) for squamous cell carcinoma of the head and neck is an established anti-cancer therapy that, by combining a photosensitizing agent (PS) with light and oxygen. PDT produces highly cytotoxic reactive oxygen species, leading to selective tumor eradication. Improving tumor selectivity is a major challenge that can be addressed by using a new generation of photosensitizing nanoparticles.

In: A Biochemical View of Head and Neck ... ISBN: 978-1-53619-370-1
Editors: D. Bartusik-Aebisher et al. © 2021 Nova Science Publishers, Inc.

Chapter 1

BIOCHEMICAL STUDIES OF HEAD CANCERS

*Lidia Bieniasz, David Aebisher, Wojciech Domka and Dorota Bartusik-Aebisher**
Medical College of The University of Rzeszów, Poland

ABSTRACT

Treatment of patients with squamous cell carcinoma of the head is a significant problem. Head cancers are among the most common cancers. Every year, more than half a million cases of squamous cell carcinoma of the head and neck are reported worldwide, mainly involving the mouth and throat, lower pharynx and larynx.

Keywords: head cancer, tumor, biochemistry

One of the greatest challenges facing modern oncology is the ability to work constantly to treat cancer. Traditional methods for diagnosis and treatment are often not precise enough to accurately map out the tumour and destroy the cancerous cells. Treating cancer is complicated due to the

---

* Corresponding Author's Email: dbartusik-aebisher@ur.edu.pl.

lifestyle and attitude of patients. The incidence of malignant neoplasms is increasing. Surgery, radiation therapy, and chemotherapy are often not sufficient cancer treatments. A thorough analysis of the processes taking place in the tumor microenvironment allowed to distinguish three stages that make up the human body's response to hostile antigens, which are tumor antigens. Therefore, Immunology is an area of cancer treatment that focuses on using the patient's immune system to fight the disease. Immunotherapy has had positive effects in many cancer patients. Head cancer is among the tumors that exhibit a strong ability to be chemo-resistant. As the name suggests, this cancer includes tumors that form in the lining of the mouth, nose, and throat area. Head cancer symptoms vary with the initial location of the tumor, but the usual symptoms are pain, ulceration, tissue involvement, and difficulties in breathing, swallowing and speech. They can also cause changes in your eyesight smell, taste, and hearing. Often, the first symptom of head cancer is enlargement of the lymph nodes in the neck, caused by the spread of the tumor into these structures. Although head and neck carcinoma rank fifth among cancer types, patient survival rates have not changed significantly over the past years (Gerberich, et al., 2020; Rubino et al., 2020; Trecca et al., 2020; Clarke et al., 2020; Bielak et al., 2020). Recent advancements in high-resolution imaging have improved the diagnostic assessment of magnetic resonance imaging (MRI) for intralabyrinthine schwannoma (ILS). This systematic review aimed to evaluate the diagnostic performance of MRI for patients. The most recently characterized genetic factors for head and neck cancer are mutations in suppressors mutations, xenobiotic metabolism enzyme genes, polymorphisms of DNA repair genes, and mutations in mitochondrial DNA. It has been observed that single-gene polymorphisms could affect treatment, whereas the coincidence of other gene mutations may increase the risk of human head and neck cancer development (Rusin et al., 2008; Mifsud et al., 2107; Workman et al., 2018; Yang et al., 2020; Li et al., 2020; Salehi et al., 2020). Head cancer has been known to physicians since antiquity. The factors and people that helped to develop the subject of head and neck surgery have been traced through history (McGurk et al., 2000; Li et al., 2020; Plath et al., 2020; Baliga et al., 2017;

Olson et al., 2018; Haapio et al., 2017; Affolter et al., 2017; Bhattasali et al., 2016; Bossi et al., 2018). Alcohol and tobacco are still a top risk factors of head and neck cancer. Other factors may influence the development of head carcinoma. To date surgery is the main treatment option, and the addition of radiotherapy following surgery is frequent for patients in the early stages of the disease. Other therapies target specific genetic molecular components connected to tumor development (Galbiatti et al., 2000; Mirabile et al., 2016; Reyes-Gibby et al., 2017; Guezennec et al., 2019; Kirke et al., 2018). Additional research is needed for a more thorough understanding of the development of head and neck carcinomas (Rodrigo et al., 2005). Recently, there has been considerable progress in molecular diagnostics in these areas. Using molecular-based technologies, it is now possible to detect cancer early in asymptomatic individuals, identify minimal residual disease at histopathologic normal surgical margins, more precisely assess tumor burden in cancer patients, and more accurately assess the prognosis of the patients (Mitchell et al., 2016; Singh et al., 2020; Nikiforov et al., 2016; Barletta et al., 2016; Gambardella et al., 2019; Machens et al., 2020; Wennerberg et al., 1993, Banda et al., 2020; Maxwell et al., 2019; Devaraja et al., 2020; Leemans et al., 2011; Rooper et al., 2018; Shaikh et al., 2017; Agaimy et al., 2018; Guo et al., 2015; Lin et al., 217; Kadeh et al., 2016; : Coca-Pelaz et al., 2015). However, despite the great promise of these new molecular approaches for cancer detection, much of the current technology limits their implementation into routine clinical use (Coca-Pelaz et al., 2018; Boon et al., 2017; Zhang et al., 2017; Lee et al., 2019; Sethi et al., 2016). The multidisciplinary team approach for the treatment of patients with head cancers has improved organization of standard clinical guidelines (Folz et al., 2008; Mowery et al., 2019; Bots et al., 2017; Patil et al., 2017; de Ridder et al., 2017). Classical diagnostic methods such as radiology and histopathology have limited sensitivities, and only by molecular techniques can minimal residual disease be detected (van Houten et al., 2000; Talwar et al., 2020; Nurminen et al. 2020; Barateau et al., 2020). Many difficulties in data interpretation are at least in part because of technical details that might have been solved by the incorporation of one or more appropriate controls. Scientist hope that this review clarifies a number of these issues and help clinicians and investigators interested in this field to understand and weigh the contradictory findings in the published studies (Kamstra et al., 2017; Chen et al., 2019; Reid et al., 2017; Gama et al., 2017). Standard therapeutic methods, surgery and radiotherapy, give good results with early stage patients, in other cases they are not satisfactory, and therapy applied poses high risk of undesirable effects. Supportive therapy allowing for the decrease in the percentage of complications is still a challenge for an oncologist. It should be conducted by an interdisciplinary team (Gleich et al., 2002; Koike et al., 2020; Frank et al., 2020; Duprez et al., 2017; Ho et al., 2018). Head cancers have multiple genetic abnormalities that influence tumor behavior and may be useful in developing new treatments. The large number of genetic changes present in head and neck cancer cells precludes meaningful use of simple molecular tests and treatments. Detection of abnormalities in multiple genes provides better prognostic information than the detection and assessment of single mutations. Head cancers comprise a complex genetic disease. Although much has been learned about the molecular genetics of head and neck cancers, continued study of multiple genes is critical for further progress. Gene therapy, although promising, must also overcome this complexity (Pignon et al., 2000). There was no significant benefit associated with adjuvant or neoadjuvant chemotherapy. Chemotherapy given concomitantly to radiotherapy gave significant benefits, but heterogeneity of the results prohibits firm conclusions (Pignon et al., 2000). Because the main meta-analysis showed only a small significant survival benefit in favour of chemotherapy, the routine use of chemotherapy is debatable. For larynx preservation, the non-significant negative effect of chemotherapy in the organ-preservation strategy indicates that this procedure must remain investigational (Pignon et al., 2000; Guevelou et al., 2019; Azzi et al., 2020; Payne et al., 2018; Coca-Pelaz et al., 2020; Zhang, 2012). Emerging evidence indicates that a small population of cancer cells is highly tumorigenic, endowed with self-renewal, and has the ability to differentiate into cells that constitute the bulk of tumors (Przybylski et al., 2018). Treating patients with squamous cell carcinoma of the head and neck is a significant problem. There is an increase in the incidence of malignant neoplasms in this region. Surgery, radiotherapy and chemotherapy are often not sufficient methods of treatment. Thorough analysis of processes occurring in the tumor microenvironment has allowed to distinguish three stages that make up the reaction of the human body to hostile antigens, which are tumor antigens. particular immunotherapy in patients with squamous cell carcinoma of the head (Yibulayin et al., 2020; Kalavrezos et al., 2020; Wada et al., 2020). There are more than half a million incident cases of squamous-cell carcinoma of the head worldwide each year, primarily affecting the oropharynx, oral cavity, hypopharynx, and larynx. New therapies are considered, along with management approaches (Haddad et al., 2008). Head squamous cell carcinoma is a major public health concern. Recent data indicate the presence of cancer stem cells in many solid tumors (Kaseb et al., 2016). Head cancers are among the 10 most frequent cancers and are the sixth most common cancers worldwide. Among these cancers, oral cavity in general and gingivobuccal complex in particular is prone to a myriad of changes with advancing age as well as a result of environmental and lifestyle-related factors (Singh, 2020; Panchappa et al., 2020; Karodpati et al., 2020; Martens et al., 2020). Measuring quality of life after head and neck cancer, is rapidly becoming the standard of care (Walshaw et al., 2020; Cohn et al., 2020; Tekin et al., 2020). Imaging surveillance is an important component of the post-treatment management of head cancers (Strauss et al., 2020). Older adults who may not complain of balance problems may nevertheless be developing subtle balance problems that may affect future functioning. This study sought to determine whether subtle problems could be predicted by standard balance testing (Cohen et al., 2020). Rhinoplasty is one of the most commonly performed aesthetic/functional procedures worldwide. Among those who seek rhinoplasty are those whose aesthetic defect is interpreted by themselves disproportionately, leading to significant suffering. They commonly have high expectations regarding the surgical outcome and are often not satisfied postoperatively (de Souza et al., 2020; Paternoster et al., 2020). Lymphomas are a heterogeneous group of malignant neoplasms of lymphocytes and their precursor cells. Lymphoma is seen 3.5% of all intraoral malignancies and is the second most common neoplasm after the squamous cell carcinoma in the head and neck region. Diffuse large B-cell lymphomas, which is a subtype of non-Hodgkin lymphoma, are seen mostly in the paraoral region (Coskunses et al., 2020). To optimize the diffusion-weighting b values and postprocessing pipeline for hybrid intravoxel incoherent motion diffusion kurtosis imaging in the head and neck region (Sijtsema et al., 2020; Wulff et al., 2020; Wada et al., 2020; Jeong et al., 2020). The entrance beam fluence of therapeutic proton scanning beams can be monitored using a gantry-attachable plastic scintillating plate. The evaluated fields were compared with reference dose maps verified by quality assurance (Jeong et al., 2020; Fernández et al., 2020; Meulemans et al., 2020; (Androjn et al., 2020; Knopf et al., 2020; Troeltzsch et al., 2020). The type of second tumor was identified as an additional independent prognosticator for DSS, with local recurrences and second primary tumors having a better prognosis than residual tumor. Increasing clinical tumor stage, increasing number of metastatic cervical lymph nodes, hypopharyngeal and supraglottic tumor location, positive section margins, and perineural invasion are identified as independent negative prognosticators for all oncologic outcome measures (Cho et al., 2020; Yu et al., 2020; Scott et al., 2020). The radiation-related complications have a tremendous impact on the quality of life. Modern radiotherapy techniques, such as intensity-modulated radiotherapy and image-guided radiotherapy, can offer precise radiation delivery and reduce the dose to the surrounding normal tissues without compromise of target coverage (Shyh-An Yeh, 2010; Gupta et al., 2020; Hosseini et al., 2020;Maroda et al., 2020; Oh et al., 2020; Zubair et al., 2020; Ehlers et al., 2020; (Mello et al., 2020; Lalonde et al., 2020; Moura et al., 2020; Ciappuccini et al., 2020; Dantas et al., 2020; Hafström et al., 2020; Cheng et al., 2020). Lipomas are common benign mesenchymal tumors that appear in the head and neck region in approximately 25% of cases where they are noted. Lipomas of the airway region are exceedingly rare, accounting for less than 1% of airway obstruction tumors (Mönnich et al., 2020; (Kim et al., 2020; Giacometti et al., 2020; Huang et al., 2020; Olin et al., 2020). Unified airway disease where upper respiratory tract inflammation including chronic rhinosinusitis affects lower airway disease is known from asthma, bronchiectasis, cystic fibrosis and primary ciliary dyskinesia (Arnda et al., 2020). Head and neck neoplasms are a relatively uniform group from the point of view of tissue structure. Changes in the genes that regulate the life processes of the cell make cancer cells acquire special characteristics. These changes determine the continuous progression of the disease and the development of resistance to treatment. For example, genes contain information, the misreading of which causes excessive formation of substances that stimulate the growth of various tissues and the multiplication of their receptors. Genes that regulate programmed natural cell death can also be damaged, thereby immortalizing the tumor cell. Typical squamous cell carcinomas of the head and neck organs are characterized by local growth, frequent metastases to nearby lymph nodes, and relatively rare distant metastases (Fu et al., 2020; Tulaci et al., 2020; Nieminen et al., 2020). In recent years, it has been shown that a certain group of squamous cell carcinomas with a different course, mainly located in the oropharyngeal region, have a causal relationship with human papillomavirus infection. These types of cancers, common in younger age groups, have a different set of gene abnormalities, typically more atypical cells, early lymph node metastases in the neck, but also higher susceptibility to radiation and chemotherapy and an overall better prognosis (Carenzo et al., 2020; Yi et al., 2020). Another specific group of head neoplasms is nasopharyngeal carcinoma. They do not have a causal relationship with the risk factors of typical squamous cell carcinomas and are common in younger people. In terms of tissue structure, there are keratinizing carcinomas, non-keratinizing carcinomas and undifferentiated carcinomas. Especially the last two subgroups of nasopharyngeal carcinomas are characterized by rapid local growth, very early metastases to the regional lymph nodes and frequent distant metastases (Carenzo et al., 2020; Yi et al., 2020). Another epithelial neoplasms affecting the head and neck organs are glandular carcinomas. They are formed from the glandular epithelium of the ducts of large and small salivary glands. In general, they are characterized by local growth, rare metastases to regional lymph nodes, while distant metastases are relatively frequent in some tissue subtypes. Glandular carcinomas of the head and neck organs are not very sensitive to radiation and chemotherapy. Rare epithelial neoplasms of the head and neck organs include small cell neuroendocrine carcinomas (which release substances such as hormones) and anaplastic carcinomas. In terms of the head and neck organs, neoplasms of non-epithelial origin, specific to the location, such as olfactory neuroma, paraganglioma and enameloma are also found. There are also non-epithelial neoplasms not specific to this area, such as soft tissue and bone sarcomas and lymphomas, which require treatment typical of such a diagnosis. Standard methods of treating patients with head and neck cancers include surgery and radiotherapy. Ideally, surgical treatment should be carried out by teams of different specialists, ensuring, apart from oncologically correct tumor removal, also the possibility of functional and aesthetic reconstruction of tissue defects. Today, radiotherapy should be carried out using modern technologies, such as conformal 3D irradiation (irradiation in which the shape of the irradiated field is precisely adapted to the shape of the tumor by means of three-dimensional treatment planning based on imaging studies) or beam intensity modulated irradiation which provides the currently optimal protection of normal tissues. Surgery and radiation therapy are often used together as a combination therapy, with the usual sequence being irradiation to supplement surgery. Chemotherapy in patients with head and neck cancer can be used in two ways. In curative treatment, chemotherapy is combined with irradiation (most often with the concomitant use of a drug called cisplatin), and in advanced cases, with the intention of increasing the likelihood of local cure, including as another option to prevent mutilating surgery. Studies have unequivocally demonstrated that in such a situation, simultaneous chemoradiotherapy is more effective than radiotherapy alone, although at the cost of increased side effects. However, this option is indicated only for patients in good general condition and without additional diseases. Another option for combination therapy is the addition of initial chemotherapy prior to concurrent chemoradiotherapy, which is especially important in cases of massive neck lymph node metastases. Chemotherapy can also be used as a standalone treatment to alleviate symptoms in patients with inoperable relapses or distant metastases. The standard chemotherapy regimen consists of 2 drugs that kill cancer cells: cisplatin and 5-fluorouracil. In patients with a worse general condition, treatment with another drug called methotrexate may be considered. In recent years, new drugs that directly damage cancer cells have also been introduced into treatment. The first of these drugs - cetuximab - is used simultaneously with radiotherapy or together with chemotherapy in case of relapse or distant metastases. The natural course of neoplastic disease of the head and neck organs and the treatment for this reason have, especially in advanced cases, an extremely negative impact on the quality of life. Patients undergoing removal of the larynx require intensive rehabilitation by a specialist in phoniatrics with the intention of developing esophageal speech and constant psychological assistance due to the effects of loss of voice function. Currently, the number of mutilating procedures performed, including laryngeal removal, has been reduced as a result of the routine use of organ-sparing treatments. Moreover, in recent years there has been a spectacular progress in the field of restorative surgery techniques, which enables the immediate reconstruction of even extensive tissue defects, which translates into an improvement in the cosmetic and functional effect. The head and neck organs, including lymph node surgery, require systematic, intensive physical rehabilitation, including the functions of the upper limbs. Rehabilitation should also apply to patients with intense late radiation reactions, which are usually irreversible and, in extreme cases, require the assistance of a surgeon. For example, tissue fibrosis after radiotherapy causes a loss of their elasticity, which in turn translates into disturbances in the functions of the head and neck organs, as well as the upper limbs. Another typical example is the drying out of the mucosa (xerostomia) as a result of damage to the secretory function of the salivary glands. This phenomenon, in addition to the patient's discomfort and difficulties in eating, causes dental problems and increasing susceptibility to recurring infections. In such situations, patients must systematically use specialist dental care. However, the basic method of limiting the severity of radiation reactions is technological progress in radiotherapy, one of the main goals of which is to improve the protection of healthy tissues. The effects of oncological treatment that require implementation of rehabilitation measures increase in proportion to the stage of cancer at the time of diagnosis. Therefore, it is important to strive to detect neoplasms at the earliest stages of development. The basic strategy to reduce the incidence of the most common, typical squamous cell carcinomas of the head and neck is to promote non-smoking, which is the strongest risk factor for cancer development in cancers of the respiratory system and upper gastrointestinal tract. The reduction in the number of smokers should translate, to the greatest extent, into a reduction in the incidence of cancers of the larynx, oral and laryngeal pharynx and oral cavity. Another important factor is high-percentage alcohol. Limiting alcohol consumption should result in a decrease in the incidence of cancers of the oral cavity, as well as cancers of the oral and laryngeal parts of the throat. It is also important to promote care for oral hygiene. Early diagnosis of head and neck cancers is extremely important. This is because it is associated with greater effectiveness, fewer side effects of the treatment and the beneficial effect of the treatment.

MILESTONES – SUMMARY

- 1500 year head and neck prosthetics
- 1597 facial plastic surgery
- 1664 cauterry glossectomy
- 1836 median mandibulotomy
- 1850 cell theory
- 1885 tissue culture
- 1896 x rays
- 1898 contrast radiotherapy
- 1902 cervical lymphatics
- 1906 radical neck dissection
- 1928 pap smear
- 1932 composite resection

- 1957 Atlas of Head and neck Surgery
- 1977 clonogenic Cell Assay

There is multiple head and neck cancers each with its own characteristics pathogenesis.

CONCLUSION

Head cancer is a collective name for all cancers located in the head and neck area except for eye, brain, ear and esophagus cancers. They usually start developing in the epithelial cells that line the moist, mucosal areas inside the head, such as inside the mouth, nose, and throat.

REFERENCES

Affolter, A., Samosny, G., Heimes, A. S., Schneider, J., Weichert, W., Stenzinger, A., Sommer, K., Jensen, A., Maye, A., Brenner, W., Mann, W. J., Brieger, J. Multikinase inhibitors sorafenib and sunitinib as radiosensitizers in head and neck cancer cell lines. *Head Neck*, 2017, 39(4):623-632.

Agaimy A, Weichert W, Haller F, Hartmann A. Diagnostische und prädiktive and neck. *Mod Pathol*. 2017 Jan; 30(s1):S104-S111.

Androjna, S., Marcius, V. Z., Peterlin, P., Strojan, P. Assessment of set-up errors in the radiotherapy of patients with head and neck cancer: standard vs. individual head suport. *Radiol Oncol,* 2020; 54(3): 364–370.

Arndal, E., Sørensen, A. L., Lapperre, T. S., Said, N., Trampedach, C., Aanæs, K., Alanin, M. C., Christensen, K. B., Backer, V., von Buchwald, C. Chronic rhinosinusitis in COPD: A prevalent but unrecognized comorbidity impacting health related quality of life. *Respir Med.,* 2020; 171, 106092.

Baliga, S., Kabarriti, R., Ohri, N., Haynes-Lewis, H., Yaparpalvi, R., Kalnicki, S., Garg, M. K. Stereotactic body radiotherapy for recurrent head and neck cancer: A critical review. *Head Neck*, 2017, 39(3):595-601.

Barateau, A., De Crevoisier, R., Largent, A., Mylona, E., Perichon, N., Castelli, J., Chajon, E., Acosta, O., Simon, A., Nunes, J. C., Lafond, C. Comparison of CBCT-based dose calculation methods in head and neck cancer radiotherapy: from Hounsfield unit to density calibration curve to deep learning. *Med Phys*, 2020. Online ahead of print.

Barletta JA, Wenig BM, Al Ghuzlan A, Kakudo K, Giordano TJ, Alves VA, Khanafshar, Bhattasali, O., Holliday, E., Kies, M. S., Hanna, E. Y., Garden, A. S., Rosenthal, D. I., Morrison, W. H., Gunn, G. B., Fuller, C, D., Zhu, X. R., Frank, S. J. Definitive proton radiation therapy and concurrent cisplatin for unresectable head and neck adenoid cystic carcinoma: A series of 9 cases and a critical review of the literature. *Head Neck*, 2016, 38 Suppl 1:E1472-80.

Bielak, L., Wiedenmann, N., Berlin, A., Nicolay, N. H., Gunashekar, D. D., Hägele, L., Lottner, T., Grosu, A. L., Bock, M. Convolutional neural networks for head and neck tumor segmentation on 7-channel multiparametric MRI: a leave-one-out analysis. *Radiat Oncol*, 2020; 15(1).

Boon, E., van der Graaf, W. T. A., Gelderblom, H., Tesselaar, M. E. T., van Es, R. J. J., Oosting, S. F., de Bree, R., van Meerten, E., Hoeben, A., Smeele, L. E., Willems, S. M., Witjes, M. J. H., Buter, J., Baatenburg de Jong, R. J., Flucke, U. E., Peer, P. G. M., Bovée, J. V. M. G., Van Herpen, C. M. L. Impact of chemotherapy on the outcome of osteosarcoma of the head and neck in adults. *Head Neck*, 2017; 39(1):140-146.

Bossi, P., Miceli, R., Benasso, M., Corvò, R., Bacigalupo, A., Sanguineti, G., Fallai, C., Merlano, M. C., Infante, G., Dani, C., Di Giannantonio, V., Licitra, L. Impact of treatment expertise on the outcome of patients with head and neck cancer treated within 6 randomized trials. *Head Neck*, 2018; 40(12):2648-2656.

Bots, W. T. C., van den Bosch, S., Zwijnenburg, E. M., Dijkema, T., van den Broek, G. B., Weijs, W. L. J., Verhoef, L. C. G., Kaanders, J. H. A. M. Reirradiation of head and neck cancer: Long-term disease control and toxicity. *Head Neck*, 2017; 39(6):1122-1130.

Calcitonin negative Medullary Thyroid Carcinoma: a challenging diagnosis or a cancer: United Kingdom National Multidisciplinary Guidelines. *J Laryngol Otol.*

Capua F, Di Martino S, Romano RM, Fiore L, Conzo A, Conzo G, Docimo G. carbohydrate and salt consumption with esophageal cancer risk: a systematic carcinoma: A comprehensive update. *Life Sci.* 2020 Mar 15; 245:117383.

Carenzo, A., Serafini, M. S., Roca, E., Paderno, A., Mattavelli, D., Romani, C., Saintigny, P., Koljenović, S., Licitra, L., De Cecco, L., Bossi, P. Gene Expression Clustering and Selected Head and Neck Cancer Gene Signatures Highlight Risk Probability Differences in Oral Premalignant Lesions. *Cells*, 2020; 9(8):1828.

chemotherapy and radiotherapy in head and neck cancer. *Anticancer Res.* 1993 Nov-.

Chen, T. H., Chang, P. M. H., Yang, M. H. Novel immune-modulating drugs for advanced head and neck cancer. *Head Neck*, 2019, 39(1):160-169.

Cheng, Z., Carobbio, A. L. C., Soggiu, L., Migliorini, M., Guastini, L., Mora, F., Fragale, M., Ascoli, A., Africano, S., Caldwell, D. G., Canevari, F. R. M., Parrinello, G., Peretti, G., Mattos, L. S. SmartProbe: a bioimpedance sensing system for head and neck cancer tissue detection. *Physiol Meas*, 2020; 41(5):054003.

Cho, S. J., Choi, B. S., Bae, Y. J., Jae-Jin Song, Ja-Won Koo, Ji-Soo Kim, Sung Hyun Baik, Sunwoo, L., Kim, J. H. Diagnostic assessment of magnetic resonance imaging for patients with intralabyrinthine schwannoma: A systematic review. *J Neuroradiol*, 2020. In Press, Corrected Proof.

Ciappuccini, R., Heutte, N., Lasne-Cardon, A., Saguet-Rysanek, V., Leroy, C., Le Hénaff, V., Vaur, D., Babin, E., Bardet, S. Tumor burden of persistent disease in patients with differentiated thyroid cancer:

correlation with postoperative risk-stratification and impact on outcome. *BMC Cancer*, 2020; 20: 765.

Clarke, J. A., Despotis, A. M., Ramirez, R. J., Zevallos, J. P., Mazul, A. L. Head and Neck Cancer Survival Disparities by Race and Rural-Urban Context. *Cancer Epidemiol Biomarkers Prev*, 2020; 29(10):1955-1961.

Coca-Pelaz A, Rodrigo JP, Triantafyllou A, Hunt JL, Rinaldo A, Strojan P, Haigentz M Jr, Mendenhall WM, Takes RP, Vander Poorten V, Ferlito A. Salivary mucoepidermoid carcinoma revisited. *Eur Arch Otorhinolaryngol.* 2015 Apr; 272(4):799-819.

Coca-Pelaz, A., Rodrigo, J. P., Suárez, C., Nixon, I. J., Mäkitie, A., Sanabria, A., Quer, M., Strojan, P., Bradford, C. R., Kowalski, L. P., Shaha, A. R., de Bree, R., Hartl, D. M., Rinaldo, A., Takes, R. P, Ferlito, A. The risk of second primary tumors in head and neck cancer: A systematic review. *Head Neck*, 2020; 42:456–466.

Coca-Pelaz, A., Takes, R. P., Hutcheson, K., Saba, N. F., Missak Haigentz J. R., Bradford, K. R., Remco de Bree, Primož Strojan, Lund, V. J., Mendenhall, W. M., Nixon, I. J., Quer, M., Rinaldo, A., Ferlito, A. Head and Neck Cancer: A Review of the Impact of Treatment Delay on Outcome. *Adv Ther. 2018*; 35(2):153-160.

Cohen, H. S., Sangi-Haghpeykar, H., Williams, S. P. Prediction of Functional Limitations in Balance after Tests of Tandem Walking and Standing Balance in Older Adults. *South Med J,* 2020; 113(9):423-426.

Cohn, J. E., Iezzi, Z., Licata, J. J., Othman, S., Zwillenberg, S. An Update on Maxillary Fractures: A Heterogenous Group. *J Craniofac Surg,* 2020, 31(7):1920-1924.

Coskunses, F. M., Cilasun, U., Topcu, P. C., Tokuc, B. Primary diffuse large B-cell lymphoma of the mandible: A case report. *Gerodontology*, 2020, 37(3):307-31.

de Lima Dantas, J. B., Martins, G. B., Lima, H. R., Carrera, M., de Almeida Reis, S. R., Medrado, A. R. Evaluation of preventive laser photobiomodulation in patients with head and neck cancer undergoing radiochemotherapy: Laser in patients with head and neck cancer. *Spec Care Dentist*, 2020; 40: 364- 373.

de Ridder, M., Klop, M., Hamming-Vrieze, O., de Boer, J. P., Jasperse, B., Smit, L., Vogel, W., van den Brekel, M., Al-Mamgani, A. Unknown primary head and neck squamous cell carcinoma in the era of fluorodeoxyglucose-positron emission tomography/CT and intensity-modulated radiotherapy. *Head Neck*, 2017; 39 (7): 1382-1391.

Duprez, F., Berwouts, D., De Neve, W., Bonte, K., Boterberg, T., Deron, P., Huvenne, W., Rottey, S., Mareel, M. Distant metastases in head and neck cancer. *Head Neck*, 2017; 39(9):1733-1743.

Ehlers, S. A., Bozanich, J. M., Arashlow, M. T., Liang, H., Nair, M. K. Large airway-obstructing retropharyngeal lipoma in an asymptomatic patient: a case report. *Int J Implant Dent*, 2020; 6: 38.

Fernández, V. E. M., Ferreiro, A. G. Acute dacryocystitis retention syndrome due to Epstein-Barr virus. *Arch Soc Esp Oftalmol*, 2020; S0365-6691(20)30323-3.

Folz, B. J., Silver, C. E., Rinaldo, A., Fagan, J. J., Pratt, L. W., Weir, N., Seitz, D., Ferlito, A. An outline of the history of head and neck oncology. *Oral Oncology*, 2008; 44(2) 2–9.

Frank, D. N., Giese, A. P. J., Hafren, L., Bootpetch, T. C., Yarza, T. K. L., Steritz, M. J., Pedro, M., Labra, P. J., Daly, K. A., Ma Leah C Tantoco, Szeremeta, W., Reyes-Quintos, M. R. T., Ahankoob, N., Llanes, E. G. D. V., Pine, H. S., Yousaf, S., Ir, D., Einarsdottir, E., de la Cruz, R. A. R., Lee, N. R., Nonato, R. M. A., Robertson, C. E., Ong, K. M. C., Magno, J. P. M., Chiong, A. N. E., Espiritu-Chiong, M. C., Luz, M., Agustin, S., Cruz, T. L. G., Abes, G. T., Bamshad, M. J., Cutiongco-de la Paz, E. M., Kere, J., Nickerson, D. A., Mohlke, K. L., Riazuddin, S., Chan, A., Mattila, P. S., Leal, S. M., Ryan, A. F., Ahmed, Z. M., Chonmaitree, T., Sale, M. M., Chiong, C. M., Santos-Cortez, R. L. P. Otitis media susceptibility and shifts in the head and neck microbiome due to SPINK5 variants. *J Med Genet*, 2020. Online ahead of print.

Galbiatti, A. L., Padovani-Junior, J. A., Maníglia, J. V., Soares Rodrigues, C. D., Pavarino, E. C., Goloni-Bertollo, E. M. Head and neck cancer: causes, prevention and treatment. *Braz J Otorhinolaryngol*. 2013; 79(2):239-47.

Gama, R. R., Song, Y., Zhang, Q., Brown, M. C., Wang, J., Habbous, S., Tong, L., Huang, S. H., O'Sullivan, B., Waldron, J., Xu, W., Goldstein, D., Liu, G. Body mass index and prognosis in patients with head and neck cancer. *Head Neck*, 2017; 39(6):1226-1233.

Gambardella C, Offi C, Patrone R, Clarizia G, Mauriello C, Tartaglia E, Di Gerberich, A. J., Attilio, M. R., Svoboda, A. Revisiting same day administration of pegfilgrastim in the age of biosimilars: A review of literature. *J Oncol Pharm Pract*, 2020. Online ahead of print.

Giacometti, V., Hounsell, A. R., McGarry, C. K. A review of dose calculation approaches with cone beam CT in photon and proton therapy. *Phys Med.*, 2020; 76: 243-276.

Gleich, L. L., Salamone, F. N. Molecular genetics of head and neck cancer. *Cancer Control*, 2002; 9(5): 369-78.

Gokce Tulaci, K., Arslan, E., Tulaci, T., Yazici, H. Which one is favorable in the elderly? Transoral rigid laryngoscopy or transnasal flexible fiberoptic laryngoscopy. *Am J Otolaryngol*, 2020; 41(6):102660.

Guevelou, J. L., Lebars, S., Kammerer, E., de Gabory, L., Vergez, S., Janot, F., Baujat, B., Righini, C., Jegoux, F., Dufour, X., Merol, J. C., Mauvais, O., Cardon, A. L., Selleret, L., Thariat, J. Head and neck cancer during pregnancy. *Head Neck*, 2019; 41(10):3719-3732.

Guezennec, C., Robin, P., Orlhac, F., Bourhis, D., Delcroix, O., Gobel, Y., Rousset, J., Schick, U., Salaün, P. Y., Abgral, R. Prognostic value of textural indices extracted from pretherapeutic 18-F FDG-PET/CT in head and neck squamous cell carcinoma. *Head Neck*, 2019, 41(2):495-502.

Gui-Ming Fu, Zhao-Hui Wang, Yi-Bo Chen, Chun-Hua Li, Yue-Jia Zhang, Xiao-Jing Li, Quan-Xin Wan. Analysis of Risk Factors for Lymph Node Metastases in Elderly Patients with Papillary Thyroid Micro-Carcinoma. *Cancer Manag Res*, 2020; 12:7143-7149.

Gupta, A. K., Love, R. P., True, R. H., Harris, J. A. Follicular Unit Excision Punches and Devices. *Dermatol Surg*, 2020. Publish Ahead of Print.

Haapio, E., Kinnunen, I., Airaksinen, J. K. E., Irjala, H., Kiviniemi, T. Excessive intravenous fluid therapy in head and neck cancer surgery. *Head Neck*, 2017, 39(1):37-41.

Haddad, R. I., Shin, D, M. Recent Advances in Head and Neck Cancer. *N Engl J Med*, 2008; 359 (11): 1143-54.

Hafström, A., Nateghi-Gillberg, B., Nilsson, M. A., Greiff, L . Patients with cutaneous head and neck melanoma, particularly elderly with more advanced primary tumors, seem to benefit from initial CT staging before considering a sentinel lymph node biopsy. *Acta Otolaryngol*, 2020; 140(9):795-802.

Ho, J. C., Phan, J. Reirradiation of head and neck cancer using modern highly conformal techniques. *Head Neck*, 2018; 40(9):2078-2093.

Hosseini, S., Schuman, T. A., Golshahi, L. Correlations to Estimate the Key Anatomical Dimensions of Pediatric Nasal Airways using Minimally Invasive Measurements of Intranasal Pressure Gradient. *J Aerosol Med Pulm Drug Deliv,* 2020. Online ahead of print.

Huang, G., Pan, S. T. ROS-Mediated Therapeutic Strategy in Chemo-/Radiotherapy of Head and Neck Cancer. *Oxid Med Cell Longev,* 2020; Volume 2020, Article ID 5047987, 30 pages.

Jagielska, B. Leczenie wspomagające w nowotworach głowy i szyi. Supportive treatment in head and neck cancer. *Onkol. Prak. Klin.* 2012; 8, 5: 189–196.

Jeong, S., Yoon, M., Chung, K., Ahn, S. H., Lee, B., Seo, J. *Clinical application of a gantry-attachable plastic scintillating plate dosimetry system in pencil beam scanning proton therapy beam monitoring,* 2020; 77:181-186.

Kalavrezos, N., Sinha, D. Head and neck sarcomas in adulthood: current trends and evolving management concepts. *Br J Oral Maxillofac Surg,* 2020; 58(8): 890-897.

Kamstra, J. I., van Leeuwen, M., Roodenburg, J. L. N., Dijkstra, P. U. Exercise therapy for trismus secondary to head and neck cancer: A systematic review. *Head Neck*, 2017; 39(1):160-169.

Karodpati, N. Clinico pathological analysis of change in voice in Indian population. *Head Neck Cancer Res*, 2020, pp. 11.

Kaseb et al., Identification, expansion and characterization of cancer cells with stem cell properties from head and neck squamous cell carcinomas. *Exp Cell Res*. 2016; 348(1): 75–86.

Kim, J. H., Choi, K. Y., Lee, S. H., Lee, D. J., Park, B. J., Yoon, D. Y., Rho, Y. S. The value of CT, MRI, and PET-CT in detecting retropharyngeal lymph node metastasis of head and neck squamous cell carcinoma. *BMC Med Imaging*, 2020; 88.

Kirke, D. N., Qureshi, M. M., Kamran, S. C., Ezzat, W., Jalisi, S., Andrew Salama, Peter C Everett, Minh Tam Truong. Role of adjuvant chemoradiotherapy in T4N0 stage IV head and neck cancer: A National Cancer Database analysis. *Head Neck*, 2018, 40:1174–1184.

Knopf, A., Jacob, S., Bier, H., Scherer, E. Q. Bilateral versus ipsilateral neck dissection in oral and oropharyngeal cancer with contralateral cN0 neck. *Eur Arch Otorhinolaryngol*, 2020; 277(11): 3161–3168.

Koike, Y., Anetai, Y., Takegawa, H., Ohira, S., Nakamura, S., Tanigawa, N. Deep learning-based metal artifact reduction using cycle-consistent adversarial network for intensity-modulated head and neck radiation therapy treatment planning. *Phys Med*. 2020; 78: 8-14.

Lalonde, A., Winey, B. A., Verburg, J. M., Paganetti, H., Sharp, G. C. Evaluation of CBCT scatter correction using deep convolutional neural networks for head and neck adaptive proton therapy. *Phys Med Biol*, 2020. Accepted Manuscript online.

Lee, J. W., Ban, M. J., Park, J. H., Lee, S. M. Visceral adipose tissue volume and CT-attenuation as prognostic factors in patients with head and neck cancer. *Head Neck*, 2019, 41(6):1605-1614.

Leemans CR, Braakhuis BJ, Brakenhoff RH. The molecular biology of head and Li, W., Chen, Y., Nie, X. Regulatory Mechanisms of lncRNAs and Their Target Gene Signaling Pathways in Laryngeal Squamous Cell Carcinoma. *Front Pharmacol*, 2020, 11:1140.

Li, X., Guo, K., Feng, Y., Guo, Y. Analysis of chemotherapy effect on the second primary malignancy for head and neck cancer patients by a nomogram based on SEER database. *Cancer Med.*, 2020, 00:1–14.

Lin MC, Lin JJ, Hsu CL, Juan HF, Lou PJ, Huang MC. GATA3 interacts with and Machens A, Lorenz K, Dralle H. Prediction of biochemical cure in patients marker in differentiated thyroid cancer - clinical considerations. *Acta Clin.*

Maroda, A. J., Spence, M. N., Larson, S. R., Estepp, J. H., Gillespie, M. B., Harris, A. J., Mamidala, M. P., Sheyn, A. M. Screening for Obstructive Sleep Apnea in Children With Sickle Cell Disease: A Pilot Study. *Laryngoscope*, 2020; 00:1–7.

Martens, R. M., Koopman, T., Noij, D. P., Pfaehler, E., Übelhör, C. M., Sharma, S., Vergeer, M. R., Leemans, C. R., Hoekstra, O. S., Yaqub, M., Zwezerijnen, G. R., Heymans, M. W., Carel F W Peeters, Remco de Bree, Pim de Graaf, Jonas A Castelijns, Ronald Boellaard. Predictive value of quantitative 18 F-FDG-PET radiomics analysis in patients with head and neck squamous cell carcinoma. *EJNMMI Res,* 2020; 10: 102.

Maxwell C, Sipos JA. *Clinical Diagnostic Evaluation of Thyroid Nodules.* May; 42(5):665-671.

McGurk, M., Goodger N. M. Head and neck cancer and its treatment: historical review. British Journal of Oral & Maxillofacial Surgery. *British Journal of Oral and Maxillofacial Surgery*, 2000; 38 (3): 209–220.

Mello, A. T., Borges, D. S., de Lima, L. P., Pessini, J., Kammer, P. V., Trindade, E B S M. Effect of oral nutritional supplements with or without nutritional counselling on mortality, treatment tolerance, and quality of life in head and neck cancer patients receiving (chemo)radiotherapy: a systematic review and meta-analysis. *Br J Nutr*, 2020; 1-18.

Meulemans, J., Debacker, J., Demarsin, H., Vanclooster, C., Neyt, P., Mennes, T., Vauterin, T., Huvenne, W., Laenen, A., Delaere, P., Poorten, V. V. Oncologic Outcomes After Salvage Laryngectomy for Squamous Cell Carcinoma of the Larynx and Hypopharynx: A Multicenter Retrospective Cohort Study. *Ann Surg Oncol*, 2020. Online ahead of print.

Mifsud, M., Eskander, A., Irish, J., Gullane, P., Gilbert, R., Brown, D., de Almeida, J. R., Urbach, D. R., Goldstein, D. P. Evolving trends in head and neck cancer epidemiology: Ontario, Canada 1993-2010. *Head Neck*, 2017, 39(9):1770-1778.

Mirabile, A., Vismara, C., Crippa, F., Bossi, P., Locati, L., Bergamini, C., Granata, R., Resteghini, C., Conte, E., Morelli, D., Scarpellini, P., Licitra, L. Health care-associated infections in patients with head and neck cancer treated with chemotherapy and/or radiotherapy. *Head Neck*, 2016, 38 Suppl 1:E1009-13.

Mönnich, D., Winter, J., Nachbar, M., Künzel, L., Boeke, S., Gani, C., Dohm, O., Zips, D., Thorwarth, D. Quality assurance of IMRT treatment plans for a 1.5 T MR-linac using a 2D ionization chamber array and a static solid phantom. *Phys Med Biol*, 2020; 65(16): 16NT01.

Moura, R. N., Arantes, V. N., Ribeiro, T. M. L., Guimarães, R. G., de Oliveira, J. F., Kulcsar, M. A. V., Sallum, R. A. A., Ribeiro-Junior, U., Maluf-Filho, F. Does a history of head and neck cancer affect outcome of endoscopic submucosal dissection for superficial esophageal squamous cell carcinoma? *Endosc Int Open*, 2020; 08: E900–E910.

Mowery, A. J., Conlin, M. J., Clayburgh, D. R. Elevated incidence of head and neck cancer in solid organ transplant recipients. *Head Neck,* 2019; 41:4009–4017.

Nair S, Chaturvedi P. The impact of peritumoral depapillation in cancers of the neck cancer. *Nat Rev Cancer*. 2011 Jan; 11(1):9-22.

Neuroendocrine Differentiation in Head and Neck Tumors. *Am J Surg Pathol*. 2018.

Nieminen, M., Aro, K., Mäkitie, A., Harlin, V., Kainulainen, S., Jouhi, L., Atula, T. Challenges in diagnosing head and neck cancer in primary health care. *Ann Med.,* 2020; 53(1):26-33.

Nikiforov YE, Seethala RR, Tallini G, Baloch ZW, Basolo F, Thompson LD, Nikiforova MN, Nosé V, Papotti M, Poller DN, Sadow PM, Tischler AS, Tuttle RM, Nurminen, J., Velhonoja, J., Heikkinen, J., Happonen, T., Nyman, M., Irjala, H., Soukka, T., Mattila, K., Hirvonen, J. Emergency neck MRI: feasibility and diagnostic accuracy in cases of neck infection. *Acta Radiol*, 2020; 284185120940242.

Oh, C. H., Lee, C. H., Kim, S. Y., Lee, S. Y., Jun, H. H., Lee, S. A family of Melnick-Needles syndrome: a case report. *BMC Pediatr*, 2020; 20(1):391.

Olin, A. B., Hansen, A. E., Rasmussen, J. H., Ladefoged, C. N., Berthelsen, A. K., Håkansson, K., Vogelius, I. R., Specht, L., Gothelf, A. B., Kjaer, A., Fischer, B. M., Andersen, F. L. Feasibility of Multiparametric Positron Emission Tomography/Magnetic Resonance Imaging as a One-Stop Shop for Radiation Therapy Planning for Patients with Head and Neck Cancer. *Int J Radiat Oncol Biol Phys*, 2020; In Press, Corrected Proof.

Olson, M. D., Van Abel, K. M., Wehrs, R. N., Garcia, J. J., Moore, E. J. Ewing sarcoma of the head and neck: The Mayo Clinic experience. *Head Neck*, 2018, 40(9):1999-2006.

Ozturk, C., Ozturk, C. N., Platek, M., Soucise, A., Laub, P., Morin, N., Lohman, R., Moon, W. Management of Expander- and Implant-Associated Infections in Breast Reconstruction. *Aesthetic Plast Surg*, 2020. Online ahead of print.

Panchappa, S. A., Jeyabalan K, A. A clinicopathological study on laryngeal cancer. *Head Neck Cancer Res*, 2020, pp. 007.

Paternoster, G., Haber, S. E., Britto, J. A., Benderbous, D., James, S., Legros, C., Khonsari, R. H., Arnaud, E. Strategy for Bone Conservation in the Two-Stage Correction of Hypertelorism in Craniofrontonasal Dysplasia. *J Craniofac Surg*, 2020; 31(6):1841-1843.

Patil, V. M., Noronha, V., Joshi, A., Ramaswamy, A., Dhumal, S., Juvekar, S., Arya, S., Mahajan, Chaturvedi, P., D'Cruz, A., Bhattacharjee, A., Prabhash, K. Neoadjuvant chemotherapy in geriatric head and neck cancers. *Head Neck*, 2017, 39(5):886-892.

Payne, K., Spruce, R., Beggs, A., Sharma, N., Kong, A., Martin, T., Parmar, S., Praveen, P., Nankivell, P., Mehanna, H. Circulating tumor DNA as a biomarker and liquid biopsy in head and neck squamous cell carcinoma. *Head Neck*, 2018; 40(7):1598-1604.

Pervej, K., Singh, M., Singh, B., Kumar, R., Singh, K., Singh, A. A clinico-pathological study of squamous cell carcinoma of gingivobuccalcomplex in Punjab. *Head Neck Cancer Res*, 2018; 7(13); 1602-1606.

Pignon, J. P., Bourhis, J., Domenge, C., Designé, L. Chemotherapy added to locoregional treatment for head and neck squamous-cell carcinoma: three meta-analyses of updated individual data. MACH-NC Collaborative Group. Meta-Analysis of Chemotherapy on Head and Neck Cancer. *Lancet*, 2000 Mar 18;355(9208):949-55.

Plath, M., Gass, J., Hlevnjak, M., Li, Q., Feng, B., Hostench, X. P., Bieg, M., Schroeder, L., Holzinger, D., Zapatka, M., Freier, K., Weichert, W., Hess, J., Zaoui, K. Unraveling most abundant mutational signatures in head and neck cancer. *Int J Cancer*, 2020, 1–13.

Przybylski, K., Majchrzak, E., Weselik, L., Golusiński, W. Immunotherapy of head and necksquamouscell carcinoma (HNSCC). Immune checkpoint blockade. *Otolaryngol Pol* 2018; 72 (6): 10-16.

Reid, P. A., Wilson, P., Li, Y., Marcu, L. G., Bezak, E. Current understanding of cancer stem cells: Review of their radiobiology and role in head and neck cancers. *Head Neck*, 2017; 39(9):1920-1932.

Reyes-Gibby, C. C., Melkonian, S. C., Hanna, E. Y., Sai-Ching J Yeung, Lu, C., Chambers, M. S., Banala, S. R., Gunn, G. B., Shete, S. S. Cohort study of oncologic emergencies in patients with head and neck cancer. *Head Neck*, 2017, 39(6):1195-1204.

Rodrigo, J. P., Ferlito, A., Carlos Sua´rez, MD, Ashok R. Shaha, MD, FACS, Carl E. Silver, MD, FACS, Kenneth O. Devaney, MD, JD, FCAP, Patrick J. Bradley, MB, BCh, BAO, DCH, MBA, FRCSI, FRCSEd, FRCS, 7 Jennifer M. Bocker, MD, Kathryn M. McLaren, BSc, MB ChB, FRCPath, FRCPE, FRCSEd, Reidar Gre´nman, MD, PhD, Alessandra Rinaldo, MD. New molecular diagnostic methods in head and neck cancer. Wiley Periodicals, *Inc. Head Neck*, 2005; 27(11): 995– 1003.

Rooper LM, Bishop JA, Westra WH. INSM1 is a Sensitive and Specific Marker of Rubino, F., Martinez-Perez, R., Vieira, S., Voscoboinik, D. S., Mural, M., Orr, A. J., Douglas A Hardesty, Ricardo L Carrau, Daniel M Prevedello. Granular cell tumors of the sellar region: what should be done after subtotal resection? A systematic review. *Pituitary*, 2020; 23(6):721-732.

Rusin, P., Markiewicz, Ł., Majsterek, I. Uwarunkowania genetyczne nowotworów głowy i szyi [Genetic predeterminations of head and neck cancer]. *Postepy Hig Med Dosw*. 2008; 62: 490-501.

Salehi, P. P., Jacobs, D., Suhail-Sindhu, T., Judson, B. L., Azizzadeh, B., Lee, Y. H. Consequences of Medical Hierarchy on Medical Students, Residents, and Medical Education in Otolaryngology. *Otolaryngol Head Neck Surg*, 2020, 163(5):906-914.

Scott, S. E., Oakley, R., Møller, H., Warburton, F. Tracking cancer occurrence in the 5 years after referral for suspected head and neck cancer. *Oral Oncol*, 2020; 109, 104955.

Sethi, N., MacLennan, K., Wood, H. M., Rabbitts, P. Past and future impact of next-generation sequencing in head and neck cancer. *Head Neck*, 2016, 38 Suppl 1:E2395-402.

Shaikh MH, Khan AI, Sadat A, Chowdhury AH, Jinnah SA, Gopalan V, Lam AK, Shyh-An Yeh. Radiotherapy for Head and Neck Cancer. *Semin Plast Surg*. 2010, 24(2): 127 136.

Sijtsema, N. D., Petit, S. F., Poot, D. H. J., Verduijn, G. M., van der Lugt, A., Hoogeman, M. S., Hernandez-Tamames, J. A. An optimal acquisition and post-processing pipeline for hybrid IVIM-DKI in head and neck. *Magn Reson Med.*, 2020. Online ahead of print.

Singh A, Singhavi H, Sathe P, Mair M, Qayyumi B, Shetty R, Bal M, Joshi P, stabilizes HIF-1α to enhance cancer cell invasiveness. *Oncogene*. 2017 Jul.

Strauss, S. B., Aiken, A. H., Lantos, J. E., Phillips, C. D. Best Practices for Post-Treatment Surveillance Imaging in Head and Neck Cancer: Application of the Neck Imaging Reporting and Data System (NI-RADS). AJR Am J Roentgenol, 2020. Online ahead of print. *Surg Oncol Clin N Am*. 2015 Jul; 24(3):397-407.

Talwar, C., McClune, A., Kelly, D., Lowe, D., Rogers, S. N. Two-week rule: suspected head and neck cancer referrals from a general medical practice perspective. *Br J Oral Maxillofac Surg,* 2020; 58(8): 981-985.

Tekin, A. M., Geert de Ceulaer, Govaerts, P., Yıldırım Bayazit, Wuyts, W., Van de Heyning, P., Topsakal, V. A New Pathogenic Variant in the TRIOBP Associated with Profound Deafness Is Remediable with Cochlear Implantation. *Audiol Neurootol*, 2020, 1-9.

Thiago Sasso Carmona de Souza, Costa Ramos de Oliveira Patrial, M. T., Correa Meneguetti, A. T., Mariana Sasso Carmona de Souza, Meneguetti, M. E., Rossato, V. T. Body Dysmorphic Disorder in Rhinoplasty Candidates: Prevalence and Functional Correlations. *Aesthetic Plast Surg*, 2020, Online ahead of print.

Trecca, E. E. C., Riggs, W. J., Mattingly, J. K., Hiss, M. M., Cassano, M., Adunka, O. F. Electrocochleography and Cochlear Implantation: A Systematic Review. *Otol Neurotol*, 2020; 41(7):864-878.

Troeltzsch, D., Niehues, S. M., Fluegge, T. V., Neckel, N., Heiland, M., Hamm, B., Shnayien, S. The diagnostic performance of perfusion CT in the detection of local tumor recurrence in head and neck cancer. *Clin Hemorheol Microcirc*, 2020; 76(2):171-177.

van Houten, V. M., Tabor, M. P., van den Brekel, M. V., Denkers, F., Wishaupt, R. G. A., Kummer, J. A., Snow, G. B., Brakenhoff, R. H. *Molecular Assays for the Diagnosis of Minimal Residual Head-and-Neck Cancer: Methods, Reliability, Pitfalls, and Solutions*, 2000; 6(10): 3803-16.

Wada, K., Hirata, T., Shinoda, Y., Teshima, T. Feasibility and effectiveness of palliative intensity-modulated radiotherapy for carotid sinus syndrome secondary to recurrent head and neck cancer. *BMJ Case Rep*, 2020; 13(6):e235066.

Wada, K., Tsuda, T., Hanada, Y., Mori, K., Nishimura, H. A Case of Ceruminous Adenocarcinoma Not Otherwise Specified (NOS) in the External Auditory Canal. *Ear Nose Throat J*, 2020. Online ahead of print.

Wall KB, LiVolsi VA, Randolph GW, Ghossein RA. Nomenclature Revision for Walshaw, E. G., Smith, M., Kanatas, A., Rogers, S. N. Handle-On-QOL: a dedicated quality of life resource following the diagnosis and treatment of head and neck cancer. *Br J Oral Maxillofac Surg*, 2020. Article in press.

Wennerberg J, Kjellén E, Lybak S, Rydell R, Pero R. Biochemical modulation of with medullary thyroid cancer. *Br J Surg*. 2020 May; 107(6):695-704.

Workman, A. D., Farquhar, D. R., Brody, R. M., Parasher, A. K., Carey, R. M., Purkey, M. T., Nagda, D. A., Brooks, J. S., Hartner, L. P., Brant, J. A., Newman, J. G. Leiomyosarcoma of the head and neck: A 17-year single institution experience and review of the *National Cancer Data Base. Head Neck*, 2018, 40(4):756-762.

Wright, C., King, D., Small, M., Gibson, C., Gardner, R., Stack Jr, B. C. The Utility of the Cl:PO4 Ratio in Patients With Variant Versions of Primary Hyperparathyroidism. *Otolaryngol Head Neck Surg*, 2020. Online ahead of print.

Wulff, N. B., Højager, A., Wessel, I., Dalton, S. O., Homøe, P. Health-Related Quality of Life Following Total Laryngectomy: A Systematic Review. *Laryngoscope*, 2020. Online ahead of print.

Yang, Y., Li, L., Zheng, Y., Liu, Q., Wei, X., Gong, X., Wang, W., Lin, P. A prospective, single-arm, phase II clinical trial of intraoperative radiotherapy using a low-energy X-ray source for local advanced Laryngocarcinoma (ILAL): a study protocol. *BMC Cancer*, 2020, 20:734.

Yi, J., Kim, T. S., Pak, J. H., Chung, J. W. Protective Effects of Glucose-Related Protein 78 and 94 on Cisplatin-Mediated Ototoxicity. *Antioxidants* (Basel), 2020; 9(8):686.

Yibulayin, F., Feng, L., Wang, M., Lu, M. M., Luo, Y., Liu, H., Yang, Z. C., Wushou, A. Head & neck acinar cell carcinoma: a population-based study using the seer registry. *BMC Cancer*, 2020. 20, Article number: 631.

Yu, S., Chen, M., Zhang, E., Wu, J., Yu, H., Yang, Z., Ma, L., Gu, X., Lu, W. Robustness study of noisy annotation in deep learning based medical image segmentation. *Phys Med Biol*, 65 (2020) 175007.

Zhang, H., Kim, S., Chen, Z., Nannapaneni, S., Chen, A. Y., Moore, C. E., Sica, G., Mosunjac, M., Nguyen, M. L. T., D'Souza, G., Carey, T. E., Peterson, L. A., McHugh, J. B., Graham, M., Komarck, C. M., Wolf, G. T., Walline, H. M., Bellile, E., Riddell, J., Pai, S. I., Sidransky, D.,

Westra, W. H., Jr, W. N. W., Lee, J. J., El-Naggar, A. K., Ferris, R. L., Seethala, R., Grandis, J. R., Chen, Z. G., Saba, N. F., Shin, D. M. Prognostic biomarkers in patients with human immunodeficiency virus-positive disease with head and neck squamous cell carcinoma. *Head Neck*, 2017, 39(12):2433-2443.

Zhang, Z., Sant'Ana Filho, M., Nör, J. E. The biology of head and neck cancer stem cells. *Oral Oncol.* 2012; 48(1): 1–9.

Zubair, F., McMahon, J., Afzali, P., Cuschieri, K., Yan, Y. S., Schipani, S., Brands, M., Ansell, M. Staging and treatment outcomes in oropharyngeal squamous cell carcinoma: a single-centre UK cohort. *Br J Oral Maxillofac Surg*, 2020. In Press, Corrected Proof.

Chapter 2

BIOCHEMICAL STUDIES OF NECK CANCERS

*Lidia Bieniasz, David Aebisher, Wojciech Domka and Dorota Bartusik-Aebisher**
Medical College of the University of Rzeszów, Rzeszów, Poland

ABSTRACT

Neck cancer is common in several regions of the World. However, most neck cancers occur in people older than 45. Neck cancer is relatively rare in women under the age of 45. Neck cancer risk is reduced by quitting smoking, and by reducing exposure to carcinogens in the environment. The most common symptom of neck cancer was difficulty breathing and stridor, followed by voice alteration and dysphagia.

Keywords: laryngeal cancer, cancer risk

Neck cancer is among the most common cancer worldwide, with a high prevalence in Asia, Brazil and Europe. Neck squamous cell carcinoma is associated with lacks of specific genetic mutations (Mitchell et al., 2016;

---

* Corresponding Author's E-mail: dbartusik-aebisher@ur.edu.pl.

Singh et al., 2020; Nikiforov et al., 2016; Maxwell et al., 2019; Gambardella et al., 2019; Banda et al., 2020; Machens et al., 2020; Wennerberg et al., 1993; McMullen et al., 2017; Lee et al., 2018; Pena et al., 2018; Marcu et al., 2019; Casbarien et al., 2013; Lucky et al., 2016; Taïeb et al., 2013; Momesso et al., 2016; Oates et al., 2008; de Luis et al., 2013; Burris et al., 2015; Cotomacio et al., 2017; de Luis et al., 2008; Chen et al., 1997; Cannataro et al., 2019; Babiuch et al. 2019; Goudet et al., 1996; Barth et al., 2010; Choi et al., 2018; Campopiano et al., 2020; Ukkonen et al., 2019; Domínguez et al., 2018; Malandrino et al., 2019; Alvarez et al., 2020; Pannone et al., 1998; de Luis DA, Izaola et al., 2007; de Luis et al., 2004 Baskaran et al., 2018; Hosseinzadeh et al., 2019). The larynx can be divided into three parts: the upper (epiglottis), middle (glottis) and lower (subglottic). Laryngeal cancer is the most common cancer of the head and neck organs. The incidence shows an upward trend (Ringash et al., 2018). It is a prospective hospital study aimed at identifying common clinical symptoms in patients with laryngeal cancer in relation to the age profile, symptomatology, disease stage, etiological factors, occupational history, histological profile and determination of treatment methods. Consumption of plant food, fruit and legumes protects against laryngeal cancer (Katabi et al., 2017; Thompson et al. 2018). Neck squamous cell carcinoma are one of the most common malignant tumors, which is prone to tumor recurrence and metastasis. At present, surgery combined with radiotherapy and chemotherapy is the conventional modality for neck squamous cell carcinoma patients, but for patients who have tumor relapse or metastasis, the treatment outcome is not ideal (Goudet et al., 1996; Barth et al., 2010; Choi et al., 2018; Campopiano et al., 2020; Ukkonen et al., 2019). The abnormality plays an important role in the development of tumor and can be used as a target of tumor diagnosis and treatment (Osai et al., 2016). Surgery including open and minimally invasive procedures is considered the standard of care for the majority of oral cavity and early larynx cancers, while radiation therapy or concurrent chemoradiation are used for the other head and neck cancers (Kaidar-Person et al., 2018; Resteghini et al., 2018; Chloupek et al., 2020). Laryngeal cancer is an abnormal and continuous growth of diseased cells in the laryngeal epithelium. Radiotherapy is a new treatment that is based on dosing and is focused on the development of evidence to guide personalisation (Mitchell et al., 2016; Singh et al., 2020; Nikiforov et al., 2016; Maxwell et al., 2019; Gambardella et al., 2019; Banda et al., 2020; Machens et al., 2020; Wennerberg et al., 1993; McMullen et al., 2017; Lee et al., 2018; Pena et al., 2018; Marcu et al., 2019; Casbarien et al., 2013; Lucky et al., 2016; Taïeb et al., 2013; Momesso et al., 2016; Oates et al., 2008; de Luis et al., 2013; Burris et al., 2015; Cotomacio et al., 2017; de Luis et al., 2008; Chen et al., 1997). Radiotherapy research discuss how exploiting these differences and taking advantage of precision medicine tools-such as genomics, radiomics, and mathematical modelling-could open new doors to personalized treatment (Caudell et al., 2017; Sim et al., 2019; Ahmad et al., 2017; Adams et al., 2006). Tumor cells exhibit elevated levels of glucose uptake, a phenomenon that has been capitalized upon for the prognostic and diagnostic imaging of a wide range of cancers using radio-labeled glucose analogs. GLUTs have been identified as rate-limiting in specific tumor. The identification and targeting of tumor-specific GLUTs provide a promising approach to block glucose-regulated metabolism and signaling more comprehensively (Adekola et al. 2012). The FLI-1 oncogene, a member of the family of transcription factors, is associated with both normal and abnormal hematopoietic cell growth and lineage-specific differentiation (Athanasiou et al., 2000). Tumor cells exhibit elevated levels of glucose uptake, a phenomenon that has been capitalized upon for the prognostic and diagnostic imaging of a wide range of cancers using radio-labeled glucose analogs (Augustin et al. 2010). Stromelysin-3 is a putative new matrix metalloproteinase which may play a role in the progression of human carcinomas, and exhibits unique structural and functional characteristics (Barbara et al., 1999; Basset et al., 1997; Basset et al., 1993). Moreover, the positive immunoreaction of all endothelial cells for CD34 is indicative of the absence of lymphatic vessels, which confirms previous ultrastructural observations (Nonogaki et al., 2010; Nozaki et al., 2006; Paran et al., 2001; Parker et al., 2004; Pavlov et al., 2009; Pawlikowski et al., 2007; Pereira et al., 1999; Podhajcer et al., 2008). Fli-1, Spi-1, and avian v-ets genes in erythroleukemia induction suggests that activation of ets gene family members plays an important role in the progression of these multistage malignancies (Beham et al., 2000; Beham et al., 1998; Ben-David et al., 1991; Białas et al., 2011). Because treatment options for vascular anomalies are widely variable and often debated, this report aims to provide a comprehensive approach to these lesions based upon current concepts and practical clinical experience (Bobik et al., 2006; Boulay et al., 2001; Bradshaw et al., 1999; Brown et al., 2010). Each patient reporting symptoms suggesting the possibility of esophageal neoplasm should, in addition to the standard medical examination undergo esophagoscopy or radiographic examination of the upper gastrointestinal tract using contrast. This division is not entirely dependent on the degree of differentiation, but rather depends on the natural course of the disease (Mitchell et al., 2016; Singh et al., 2020; Nikiforov et al., 2016; Maxwell et al., 2019; Gambardella et al., 2019; Banda et al., 2020; Machens et al., 2020; Wennerberg et al., 1993; McMullen et al., 2017; Lee et al., 2018; Pena et al., 2018; Marcu et al., 2019; Casbarien et al., 2013; Lucky et al., 2016; Taïeb et al., 2013; Momesso et al., 2016; Oates et al., 2008; de Luis et al., 2013; Burris et al., 2015; Cotomacio et al., 2017; de Luis et al., 2008; Chen et al., 1997). Salivary gland cancer is most often located in the parotid glands and twice as rarely in the submandibular glands. Lymph node metastases as well as distant metastases are rare. These tumors rarely recur, and surgery to remove the tumor usually provides a permanent cure. Lymph node metastases are rare (Ledda et al., 1997; Liang et al., 2000; Lipka et al., 2008; Lund et al., 2010; Macheda et al., 2005; Mager et al., 1998; Mai H. 2013; McClung 2007). The exception is adenocystic carcinoma, in which, often over many years, there may be slow metastases to the lungs, less often to the liver and bone (Koblinski et al., 2005; Kryvenko et al., 2013; Kukwa et al., 2011; Lastres et al., 1996; Lebrin et al., 2005). The standard treatment in patients with large salivary gland cancers is surgical excision of the organ with the intention of healing. It is worth noting that in the case of lung metastases in the course of adenocystic carcinoma, it is always advisable to consider surgical treatment, especially as the course of the disease is often slow (Hofland et al., 2003; Howard et al., 1996; Hoyer et al., 1995; Iacobuzio-Donahue et al., 2002; Ikuta et al., 2005; Itinteang et al., 2011). The prognosis for most salivary gland cancer subtypes is good provided that surgery is performed to completely remove the tumor cells. It should be noted that in many cases long-term survival does not mean a permanent cure, because relapses may occur after several or even several years, especially in the course of adenocystic carcinoma (Chlenski et al., 2004; Costello et al., 2004; Dallas et al., 2008; Dasgupta et al., 2004; Delebecq et al., 2000; Demirci et al., 2013; Ding et al., 2006; Duerr et al., 2008; Eckert., 2011; Enjolras et al., 1997; Folpe et al., 2001; Folpe et al., 2000; Fonsatti et al., 2000; Funk et al., 1993). The most important risk factor is exposure to cigarette smoke, and the disease is rare in never-smokers. Other factors include exposure to wood dust, coal dust, and inhaled chemicals (Gallot et al., 2007; Gilles et al., 1998; Grabellus et al., 2012; Greene et al., 2008; Hajdu et al., 2003). They are potent regulators of vascular development and vessel remodeling and play key roles in atherosclerosis and restenosis, regulating endothelial, smooth muscle cell, macrophage, T cell, and probably vascular calcifying cell responses (Müssig et al., 2009; Ngan et al., 2008, Nguyen et al., 2005; Nicolai et al., 2012). It contributes to restenosis by augmenting neointimal cell proliferation and collagen accumulation (Medina et al., 2002; Mercado-Pimentel et al., 2007; Muller et al., 1993; Mulliken et al., 1982; Porter et al., 1995; Prada et al., 2007; Renkonen et al., 2013; Reubi et al., 1994). Since these somatostatin receptor subtypes probably mediate distinct somatostatin actions, it may be worthwhile to search for subtype-specific analogues to use for the treatment and diagnosis of these tumors (Rio et al., 2005; Rosenblatt et al., 1997; Rumpler et al., 2003; Sage et al., 2001). It functions as a permissive reactive tumor-host microenvironment and provides sustenance for the floating tumor cells through a plethora of survival/metastasis-associated molecules (Said et al., 2007; Shi et al., 2004; Sosa et al., 2007; Sure et al., 2005; Thewes et al., 1999; Tirakotai et al., 2006; Tsujie et al., 2006; Vikkula et al., 2001; Wang et al., 2009; Watkins et al., 2005). The diagnosis of cancer of the large salivary glands may be based on the collection of cells from the tumor by means of a needle puncture, interpreted by an experienced physician. The final determination of the type of neoplasm is based on the overall evaluation of the removed tumor, and surgery is always the initial standard treatment (Watson et al., 1992; Wendler et al., 2007; Winter et al., 1996; Wolf et al., 1992; Yamashita et al., 2004; (Yang et al., 2007; Yi et al., 1997; Yu et al., 2006; Zhang et al., 1995; Zhang et al., 2011; Zhang et al., 2010). The prognosis for most salivary gland cancer subtypes is good provided that surgery is performed to completely remove the tumor cells. Long-term cure rates are then at the level of 60-80%. It should be noted that in many cases long-term survival does not mean a permanent cure, because relapses may occur after several or even several years, especially in the course of adenocystic carcinoma (Watson et al., 1992; Wendler et al., 2007; Winter et al., 1996; Wolf et al., 1992; Yamashita et al., 2004; (Yang et al., 2007; Yi et al., 1997; Yu et al., 2006; Zhang et al., 1995; Zhang et al., 2011; Zhang et al., 2010). The problem of diagnosis in the field of head and neck region is still valid. Specific diagnosis and precise estimation of the tumor's size with the use of CT and MRI imaging is generally unsatisfactory. Neck cancer cells intake large quantities of glucose and utilize it in the process of glycolysis. The oxidative phosphorylation is not efficient in the transformed cells and defects in mitochondrial functions are at the heart of malignant cell transformation. Disruption of the oxidative phosphorylation chain has been described in the neoplasms (Zou et al., 2009; Gronkiewicz et al., 2014; Czarnecka et al., 2009; Buckmiller et al., 2010; Andreassen et al., 2018).

CONCLUSION

Neck cancer cells represent a specific metabolic state. Neck cancer cells are the most common type of cancer, accounting for 90 percent or more of all laryngeal cancers. More than 70 large follow-up studies have investigated the etiology of the larynx cancer and squamous cell carcinoma.

REFERENCES

Adams D.M., Lucky A.W.: Cervicofacial vascular anomalies. I. Hemangiomas and other benign vascular tumors. *Semin. Pediatr. Surg.,* 2006; 15: 124-132.

Adekola K., Rosen S.T., Shanmugam M.: Glucose transporters in cancer metabolism. *Curr. Opin. Oncol.,* 2012; 24: 650-654.

Ahmad, P., Sana, J., Slavik, M., Slampa, P., Smilek, P., Slaby, O. Micro RNAs Involvement in Radioresistance of Head and Neck Cancer. *DisMarkers,* 2017: 8245345.

Alvarez AL, Mulder M, Handelsman RS, Lew JI, Farra JC. High Rates of Underlying Thyroid Cancer in Patients Undergoing Thyroidectomy for Hyperthyroidism. *J Surg Res.* 2020 Jan; 245:523-528.

Andreassen C.N., Eriksen J.G., Jensen K., Hansen C.R., Sørensen B.S., Lassen P., Alsner J., Schack L.M.H., Overgaard J., Grau C. IMRT - Biomarkers for dose escalation, dose de-escalation and personalized medicine in radiotherapy for head and neck cancer. *Oral Oncol, Oral Oncol,* 2018; 86:91-99.

Athanasiou M., Mavrothalassitis G., Sun-Hoffman L., Blair D.G.: FLI1 is a suppressor of erythroid differentiation in human hematopoietic cells. *Leukemia,* 2000; 14: 439-445.

Augustin R.: The protein family of glucose transport facilitators: It's not only about glucose after all. *IUBMB Life,* 2010; 62: 315-333.

Babiuch K, Bednarczyk A, Gawlik K, Pawlica-Gosiewska D, Kęsek B, Darczuk D, Stępień P, Chomyszyn-Gajewska M, Kaczmarzyk T. Evaluation of enzymatic and non-enzymatic antioxidant status and biomarkers of oxidative stress in saliva of patients with oral squamous cell carcinoma and oral leukoplakia: a pilot study. *Acta Odontol Scand.* 2019 Aug;77(6):408-418.

Banda KJ, Chiu HY, Hu SH, Yeh HC, Lin KC, Huang HC. Associations of dietary carbohydrate and salt consumption with esophageal cancer risk: a systematic review and meta-analysis of observational studies. *Nutr Rev.* 2020 Aug 1;78(8):688-698.

Barbara N.P., Wrana J.L., Letarte M.: Endoglin is an accessory protein that interacts with the signaling receptor complex of multiple members of the transforming growth factor-β superfamily. *J. Biol. Chem.*, 1999; 274: 584-594.

Barth RF, Vicente MG, Harling OK, Kiger WS 3rd, Riley KJ, Binns PJ, Wagner FM, Suzuki M, Aihara T, Kato I, Kawabata S. Current status of boron neutron capture therapy of high grade gliomas and recurrent head and neck cancer. *Radiat Oncol.* 2012 Aug 29;7:146.

Baskaran N, Selvam GS, Yuvaraj S, Abhishek A. Parthenolide attenuates 7,12-dimethylbenz[a]anthracene induced hamster buccal pouch carcinogenesis. *Mol Cell Biochem.* 2018 Mar;440(1-2):11-22.

Basset P., Bellocq J.P., Lefebvre O., Noël A., Chenard M.P., Wolf C., Anglard P., Rio M.C.: Stromelysin-3: a paradigm for stroma-derived factors implicated in carcinoma progression. *Crit. Rev. Oncol. Hematol.*, 1997; 26: 43-53.

Basset P., Wolf C., Chambon P.: Expression of the stromelysin-3 gene in fibroblastic cells of invasive carcinomas of the breast and other human tissues: a review. *Breast Cancer Res. Treat.*, 1993; 24: 185-193.

Beham A., Beham-Schmid C., Regauer S., Auböck L., Stammberger H.: Nasopharyngeal angiofibroma: true neoplasm or vascular malformation? *Adv. Anat. Pathol.*, 2000; 7: 36-46.

Beham A., Regauer S., Beham-Schmid C., Kainz J., Stammberger H.: Expression of CD34-antigen in nasopharyngeal angiofibromas. *Int. J. Pediatr. Otorhinolaryngol.*, 1998; 44: 245-250.

Ben-David Y., Giddens E.B., Letwin K., Bernstein A.: Erythroleukemia induction by Friend murine leukemia virus: insertional activation of a new member of the ets gene family, Fli-1, closely linked to c-ets-1. *Genes Dev.*, 1991; 5: 908-918.

Białas M., Papla B., Bulanda A.: Immunohistochemical investigation of selected endothelial markers in pulmonary epithelioid haemangioendothelioma. *Pol. J. Pathol.*, 2011; 62: 236-240.

Bobik A.: Transforming growth factor-βs and vascular disorders. *Arterioscler. Thromb. Vasc. Biol.*, 2006; 26: 1712-1720.

Boulay A., Masson R., Chenard M.P., El Fahime M., Cassard L., Bellocq J.P., Sautes-Fridman C., Basset P., Rio M.C.: High cancer cell death in syngeneic tumors developed in host mice deficient for the stromelysin-3 matrix metalloproteinase. *Cancer Res.*, 2001; 61: 2189-2193.

Bradshaw A.D., Francki A., Motamed K., Howe C., Sage E.H.: Primary mesenchymal cells isolated from SPARC-null mice exhibit altered morphology and rates of proliferation. *Mol. Biol. Cell*, 1999; 10: 1569-1579.

Brown J.G., Folpe A.L., Rao P., Lazar A.J., Paner G.P., Gupta R., Parakh R., Cheville J.C., Amin M.B.: Primary vascular tumors and tumor-like lesions of the kidney: a clinicopathologic analysis of 25 cases. *Am. J. Surg. Pathol.*, 2010; 34: 942-949.

Brown T.J., Shaw P.A., Karp X., Huynh M.H., Begley H., Ringuette M.J.: Activation of SPARC expression in reactive stroma associated with human epithelial ovarian cancer. *Gynecol. Oncol.*, 1999; 75: 25-33.

Buckmiller L.M., Richter G.T., Suen J.Y. Diagnosis and management of hemangiomas and vascular malformations of the head and neck. *Oral Dis.* 2010;16(5):405-18.

Buckmiller L.M., Richter G.T., Suen J.Y.: Diagnosis and management of hemangiomas and vascular malformations of the head and neck. *Oral Dis.*, 2010; 16: 405-418.

Burris J.L., Studts J.L., DeRosa A.P., Ostroff J.S. Systematic Review of Tobacco Use after Lung or Head/Neck Cancer Diagnosis: Results and Recommendations for Future Research. *Cancer Epidemiol Biomarkers Prev.* 2015 Oct;24(10):1450-61.

Campana D., Capurso G., Partelli S., Nori F., Panzuto F., Tamburrino D., Cacciari G., Delle Fave G., Falconi M., Tomassetti P.: Radiolabelled somatostatin analogue treatment in gastroenteropancreatic neuroendocrine tumours: factors associated with response and suggestions for therapeutic sequence. *Eur. J. Nucl. Med. Mol. Imaging*, 2013; 40: 1197-1205.

Cannataro V.L., Gaffney S.G., Sasaki T., Issaeva N., Grewal N.K.S., Grandis J.R., Yarbrough W.G., Burtness B., Anderson K.S., Townsend J.P. APOBEC-induced mutations and their cancer effect size in head and neck squamous cell carcinoma. *Oncogene.* 2019 May; 38(18):3475-3487.

Casbarien O., Cresta P., Silva C., Feliu M.S., Badia A., Delgado N.L., Navigante A., Slobodianik N. Specific nutritional supplement (Supportan®) in the supportive care of the radio-chemotherapy treatment of head and neck cancers: biochemical parameters. Preliminary study. *Endocr Metab Immune Disord Drug Targets.* 2013 Dec;13(4):348-50.

Caudell, J.J., Torres-Roca, J.F., Gillies, R.J., Enderling, H., Kim, S., Rishi, A., Moros, E.G., Harrison, L.B. The future of personalised radiotherapy for head and neckcancer. *Lancet Oncol,* 2017, 18(5):e266-e273.

Chen H.C., Leung S.W., Wang C.J., Sun L.M., Fang F.M., Hsu J.H. Effect of megestrol acetate and prepulsid on nutritional improvement in patients with head and neck cancers undergoing radiotherapy. *Radiother Oncol.* 1997 Apr;43(1):75-9.

Chien C.Y., Su C.Y., Hwang C.F., Chuang H.C., Chen C.M., Huang C.C.: High expressions of CD105 and VEGF in early oral cancer predict potential cervical metastasis. *J. Surg. Oncol.,* 2006; 94: 413-417.

Chlenski A., Liu S., Baker L.J., Yang Q., Tian Y., Salwen H.R., Cohn S.L.: Neuroblastoma angiogenesis is inhibited with a folded synthetic molecule corresponding to the epidermal growth factor-like module of the follistatin domain of SPARC. *Cancer Res.,* 2004; 64: 7420-7425.

Chloupek, A., Zarzycki, K., Dąbrowski, J., Domański, W. Parotid gland tumors. Results of retrospective analysis of 149 patients treated at the Clinical Department of Cranio-Maxillofacial Surgery, Clinic of Otolaryngology and Oncologic Laryngology of Military Institute of Medicine in Warsaw in years 2006-2016. *Otolaryngol Pol* 2017, 71(3):37-42.

Choi N., Park S.I., Kim H., Sohn I, Jeong H.S. The impact of unplanned reoperations in head and neck cancer surgery on survival. *Oral Oncol.* 2018 Aug;83:38-45.

Costello B., Li C., Duff S., Butterworth D., Khan A., Perkins M., Owens S., Al-Mowallad A.F., O'Dwyer S., Kumar S.: Perfusion of 99Tcm- -

labeled CD105 Mab into kidneys from patients with renal carcinoma suggests that CD105 is a promising vascular target. *Int. J. Cancer,* 2004; 109: 436-441.

Cotomacio C., Campos L., Simões A., Jaguar G., Crosato E.M., Abreu-Alves F. Influence of bethanechol on salivary parameters in irradiated patients. *Med Oral Patol Oral Cir Bucal.* 2017 Jan 1;22(1):e76-e83.

Czarnecka A.M., Kukwa W., Ścińska A., Kukwa A. Metabolic markers of head and neck tumors - clinical applications and biochemical background. *Polish Otolaryngology* 2009 (63):6, 478-484.

Dallas N.A., Samuel S., Xia L., Fan F., Gray M.J., Lim S.J., Ellis L.M.: Endoglin (CD105): a marker of tumor vasculature and potential target for therapy. *Clin. Cancer Res.,* 2008; 14: 1931-1937.

Dasgupta P.: Somatostatin analogues: multiple roles in cellular proliferation, neoplasia, and angiogenesis. *Pharmacol. Ther.,* 2004; 102: 61-85.

de Luis D.A., Izaola O., Aller R., González-Sagrado M., Cuellar L., Terroba M.C., Martín T. Influence of a W3 fatty acids oral enhanced formula in clinical and biochemical parameters of head and neck cancer ambulatory patients. *An Med. Interna 2008;*25(6):275-8.

de Luis D.A., Izaola O., Aller R., González-Sagrado M., Cuéllar L., Terroba M.C. Influencia de una fórmula enriquecida en ácidos omega 3 y arginina sobre los parámetros bioquímicos en pacientes intervenidos por cáncer de cabeza y cuello [Utility of a omega 3 fatty acids oral enhanced formula in biochemical parameters of head and neck cancer patients]. *Med Clin (Barc).* 2004 Oct 16;123(13):499-500.

de Luis D.A., Izaola O., Cuellar L., Terroba M.C., de la Fuente B., Cabezas G. A randomized clinical trial with two doses of a omega 3 fatty acids oral and arginine enhanced formula in clinical and biochemical parameters of head and neck cancer ambulatory patients. *Eur Rev Med Pharmacol Sci.* 2013.

de Luis D.A., Izaola O., Cuellar L., Terroba M.C., Martin T., Aller R. Clinical and biochemical outcomes after a randomized trial with a high dose of enteral arginine formula in postsurgical head and neck cancer patients. *Eur J Clin Nutr.* 2007 Feb; 61(2):200-4.

Delebecq T.J., Porte H., Zerimech F., Copin M.C., Gouyer V., Dacquembronne E., Balduyck M., Wurtz A., Huet G.: Overexpression level of stromelysin 3 is related to the lymph node involvement in non-small cell lung cancer. *Clin. Cancer Res.*, 2000; 6: 1086-1092.

Demirci E., Ocak M., Kabasakal L., Araman A., Ozsoy Y., Kanmaz B.: Comparison of Ga-68 DOTA-TATE and Ga-68 DOTA-LAN PET/CT imaging in the same patient group with neuroendocrine tumours: preliminary results. *Nucl. Med. Commun.*, 2013; 34: 727-732.

Ding S., Li C., Lin S., Yang Y., Liu D., Han Y., Zhang Y., Li L., Zhou L., Kumar S.: Comparative evaluation of microvessel density determined by CD34 or CD105 in benign and malignant gastric lesions. *Hum. Pathol.*, 2006; 37: 861-866.

Domínguez J.M., Martínez M.T., Massardo J.M., Muñoz S., Droppelmann N., González H.E., Mosso L. Riesgo de recurrencia en cáncer diferenciado de tiroides: escala MINSAL [Risk of recurrence in differentiated thyroid cancer]. *Rev Med Chil.* 2018 Mar;146(3):282-289.

Duerr S., Wendler O., Aigner T., Karosi S., Schick B.: Metalloproteinases in juvenile angiofibroma - a collagen rich tumor. *Hum. Pathol.*, 2008; 39: 259-268.

Eckert A.W., Lautner M.H., Schutze A., Taubert H., Schubert J., Bilkenroth U.: Coexpression of hypoxia-inducible factor-1α and glucose transporter-1 is associated with poor prognosis in oral squamous cell carcinoma patients. *Histopathology*, 2011; 58: 1136-1147.

Enjolras O.: Classification and management of the various superficial vascular anomalies: hemangiomas and vascular malformations. *J. Dermatol.*, 1997; 24: 701-710.

Folpe A.L., Chand E.M., Goldblum J.R., Weiss S.W.: Expression of Fli1, a nuclear transcription factor, distinguishes vascular neoplasms from potential mimics. *Am. J. Surg. Pathol.*, 2001; 25: 1061-1066.

Folpe A.L., Hill C.E., Parham D.M., O'Shea P.A., Weiss S.W.: Immunohistochemical detection of FLI-1 protein expression: a study of 132 round cell tumors with emphasis on CD99-positive mimics of

Ewing's sarcoma/primitive neuroectodermal tumor. *Am. J. Surg. Pathol.*, 2000; 24: 1657-1662.

Fonsatti E., Jekunen A.P., Kairemo K.J., Coral S., Snellman M., Nicotra M.R., Natali P.G., Altomonte M., Maio M.: Endoglin is a suitable target for efficient imaging of solid tumors: in vivo evidence in a canine mammary carcinoma model. *Clin. Cancer Res.*, 2000; 6: 2037-2043.

Funk S.E., Sage E.H.: Differential effects of SPARC and cationic SPARC peptides on DNA synthesis by endothelial cells and fibroblasts. *J. Cell. Physiol.*, 1993; 154: 53-63.

Gallot D., Marceau G., Laurichesse-Delmas H., Vanlieferinghen P., Dechelotte P.J., Lemery D., Sapin V.: The changes in angiogenic gene expression in recurrent multiple chorioangiomas. *Fetal Diagn. Ther.*, 2007; 22: 161-168.

Gambardella C., Offi C., Patrone R., Clarizia G., Mauriello C., Tartaglia E., Di Capua F., Di Martino S., Romano R.M., Fiore L., Conzo A., Conzo G., Docimo G. Calcitonin negative Medullary Thyroid Carcinoma: a challenging diagnosis or a medical dilemma? *BMC Endocr Disord.* 2019 May 29;19(Suppl 1):45.

Gilles C., Bassuk J.A., Pulyaeva H., Sage E.H., Foidart J.M., Thompson E.W.: SPARC/osteonectin induces matrix metalloproteinase 2 activation in human breast cancer cell lines. *Cancer Res.*, 1998; 58: 5529-5536.

Grabellus F., Nagarajah J., Bockisch A., Schmid K.W., Sheu S.Y.: Glucose transporter 1 expression, tumor proliferation, and iodine/glucose uptake in thyroid cancer with emphasis on poorly differentiated thyroid carcinoma. *Clin. Nucl. Med.*, 2012; 37: 121-127.

Greene A.K., Kim S., Rogers G.F., Fishman S.J., Olsen B.R., Mulliken J.B.: Risk of vascular anomalies with Down syndrome. *Pediatrics,* 2008; 121: e135-e140.

Gronkiewicz Z., Krzeski A., Kukwa W. Wybrane markery biologiczne w niektórych zmianach naczyniowych głowy i szyi [Selected biological markers in various vascular lesions of the head and neck]. *Postepy Hig Med Dosw (online),* 2014; 68: 1206-1215.

Hajdu I., Szentirmai E., Obal F. Jr., Krueger J.M.: Different brain structures mediate drinking and sleep suppression elicited by the somatostatin analog, octreotide, in rats. *Brain Res.,* 2003; 994: 115-123.

Hofland L.J., Lamberts S.W.: The pathophysiological consequences of somatostatin receptor internalization and resistance. *Endocr. Rev.,* 2003; 24: 28-47.

Hosseinzadeh S., Alipanah-Moghadam R., Isapanah Amlashi F., Nemati A. Evaluation of Haptoglobin Genotype and Some Risk Factors of Cancer in Patients with Early Stage Esophageal Cancer. *Asian Pac J Cancer Prev.* 2019 Oct 1;20(10):2897-2901.

Howard J.C., Berger L., Bani M.R., Hawley R.G., Ben-David Y.: Activation of the erythropoietin gene in the majority of F-MuLV-induced erythroleukemias results in growth factor independence and enhanced tumorigenicity. *Oncogene,* 1996; 12: 1405-1415.

Hoyer D., Bell G.I., Berelowitz M., Epelbaum J., Feniuk W., Humphrey P.P., O'Carroll A.M., Patel Y.C., Schonbrunn A., Taylor J.E., Reisine T.: Classification and nomenclature of somatostatin receptors. *Trends Pharmacol. Sci.,* 1995; 16: 86-88.

Iacobuzio-Donahue C.A., Argani P., Hempen P.M., Jones J., Kern S.E.: The desmoplastic response to infiltrating breast carcinoma: gene expression at the site of primary invasion and implications for comparisons between tumor types. *Cancer Res.,* 2002; 62: 5351-5357.

Ikuta Y., Nakatsura T., Kageshita T., Fukushima S., Ito S., Wakamatsu K., Baba H., Nishimura Y.: Highly sensitive detection of melanoma at an early stage based on the increased serum secreted protein acidic and rich in cysteine and glypican-3 levels. *Clin. Cancer Res.,* 2005;11: 8079-8088.

Interna. 2008 Jun;25(6):275-8. *Spanish. PMID:* 19295974.

Itinteang T., Vishvanath A., Day D.J., Tan S.T.: Mesenchymal stem cells in infantile haemangioma. *J. Clin. Pathol.,* 2011; 64: 232-236.

Kaidar-Person, O., Gil, Z., Billan, S. Precision medicine in head and neckcancer, *Drug Resist Updat,* 2018, 40:13-16.

Katabi, N., Lewis, J.S. Update from the 4th Edition of the World Health Organization Classification of Head and Neck Tumours: WhatIs New in the 2017 WHO Blue Book for Tumors and Tumor-Like Lesions of the Neck and Lymph Nodes. *Head Neck Pathol* 2017; 11(1):48-54.

Koblinski J.E., Kaplan-Singer B.R., VanOsdol S.J., Wu M., Engbring J.A., Wang S., Goldsmith C.M., Piper J.T., Vostal J.G., Harms J.F., Welch D.R., Kleinman H.K.: Endogenous osteonectin/SPARC/BM-40 expression inhibits MDA-MB-231 breast cancer cell metastasis. *Cancer Res.*, 2005; 65: 7370-7377.

Kryvenko O.N., Epstein J.I.: Testicular hemangioma: a series of 8 cases. *Am. J. Surg. Pathol.*, 2013; 37: 860-866.

Kukwa W., Andrysiak R., Kukwa A., Hubalewska-Dydejczyk A., Gronkiewicz Z., Wojtowicz P., Krolicki L., Wierzchowski W., Grochowski T., Czarnecka A.M.: 99mTC-octreotide scintigraphy and somatostatin receptor subtype expression in juvenile nasopharyngeal angiofibromas. *Head Neck,* 2011; 33: 1739-1746.

Lastres P., Letamendia A., Zhang H., Rius C., Almendro N., Raab U., López L.A., Langa C., Fabra A., Letarte M., Dernabóu C.: Endoglin modulates cellular responses to TGF-β1. *J. Cell. Biol.,* 1996; 133: 1109-1121.

Lebrin F., Deckers M., Bertolino P., Ten Dijke P.: TGF-β receptor function in the endothelium. *Cardiovasc. Res.,* 2005; 65: 599-608.

Ledda M.F., Adris S., Bravo A.I., Kairiyama C., Bover L., Chernajovsky Y., Mordoh J., Podhajcer O.L.: Suppression of SPARC expression by antisense RNA abrogates the tumorigenicity of human melanoma cells. *Nat. Med.,* 1997; 3: 171-176.

Lee D.S., O'Keefe R.A., Ha P.K., Grandis J.R., Johnson D.E. Biochemical Properties of a Decoy Oligodeoxynucleotide Inhibitor of STAT3 Transcription Factor. *Int J Mol Sci.* 2018 May 30; 19(6):1608.

Liang J., Yi Z., Lianq P.: The nature of juvenile nasopharyngeal angiofibroma. Otolaryngol. *Head Neck Surg.,* 2000; 123: 475-481.

Lipka D., Boratyński J.: Metalloproteinases. Structure and function. *Advances Hig. Med. Exp.* 2008; 62: 328-336.

Lucky S.S., Idris N.M., Huang K., Kim J., Li Z., Thong P.S., Xu R., Soo K.C., Zhang Y. In vivo Biocompatibility, Biodistribution and Therapeutic Efficiency of Titania Coated Upconversion Nanoparticles for Photodynamic Therapy of Solid Oral Cancers. *Theranostics.* 2016 Jul 18; 6(11):1844-65.

Lund V.J., Stammberger H., Nicolai P., Castelnuovo P., Beal T., Beham A., Bernal-Sprekelsen M., Braun H., Cappabianca P., Carrau R., Cavallo L., Clarici G., Draf W., Esposito F., Fernandez-Miranda J. i wsp.: European position paper on endoscopic management of tumours of the nose, paranasal sinuses and skull base. *Rhinol. Suppl.,* 2010; 48 (Suppl. 22): 1-143.

Macheda M.L., Rogers S., Best J.D.: Molecular and cellular regulation of glucose transporter (GLUT) proteins in cancer. *J. Cell. Physiol.,* 2005; 202: 654-662.

Machens A., Lorenz K., Dralle H. Prediction of biochemical cure in patients with medullary thyroid cancer. *Br J Surg.* 2020 May; 107(6):695-704.

Mager A.M., Grapin-Botton A., Ladjali K., Meyer D., Wolff C.M., Stiegler P., Bonnin M.A., Remy P.: The avian fli gene is specifically expressed during embryogenesis in a subset of neural crest cells giving rise to mesenchyme. *Int. J. Dev. Biol.,* 1998; 42: 561-572.

Mai H.M., Zheng J.W., Wang Y.A., Yang X.J., Zhou Q., Qin Z.P., Li K.L.: CD133 selected stem cells from proliferating infantile hemangioma and establishment of an in vivo mice model of hemangioma. *Chin. Med. J.,* 2013; 126: 88-94.

Malandrino P., Tumino D., Russo M., Marescalco S., Fulco R.A., Frasca F. Surveillance of patients with differentiated thyroid cancer and indeterminate response: a longitudinal study on basal thyroglobulin trend. *J Endocrinol Invest.* 2019 Oct; 42(10):1223-1230.

Marcu L.G., Boyd C., Bezak E. Feeding the Data Monster: Data Science in Head and Neck Cancer for Personalized Therapy. *J Am Coll Radiol.* 2019 Dec; 16(12):1695-1701.

Maxwell C., Sipos J.A. Clinical Diagnostic Evaluation of Thyroid Nodules. *Endocrinol Metab Clin North Am.* 2019 Mar; 48(1):61-84.

McClung H.M., Thomas S.L., Osenkowski P., Toth M., Menon P., Raz A., Fridman R., Rempel S.A.: SPARC upregulates MT1-MMP expression, MMP-2 activation, and the secretion and cleavage of galectin-3 in U87MG glioma cells. *Neurosci. Lett.,* 2007; 419: 172-177.

McMullen C., Rocke D., Freeman J. Complications of Bilateral Neck Dissection in Thyroid Cancer From a Single High-Volume Center. *JAMA Otolaryngol Head Neck Surg.* 2017 Apr 1; 143(4):376-381.

Medina R.A., Owen G.I.: Glucose transporters: expression, regulation and cancer. *Biol. Res.,* 2002; 35: 9-26.

Mercado-Pimentel M.E., Hubbard A.D., Runyan R.B.: Endoglin and Alk5 regulate epithelial-mesenchymal transformation during cardiac valve formation. *Dev. Biol.,* 2007; 304: 420-432.

Mitchell A.L., Gandhi A., Scott-Coombes D., Perros P. Management of thyroid cancer: United Kingdom National Multidisciplinary Guidelines. *J Laryngol Otol.* 2016;130(S2):S150-S160.

Muller D., Wolf C., Abecassis J., Millon R., Engelmann A., Bronner G., Rouyer N., Rio M.C., Eber M., Methlin G., Chambon P., Basset P.: Increased stromelysin 3 gene expression is associated with increased local invasiveness in head and neck squamous cell carcinomas. *Cancer Res.,* 1993; 53: 165-169.

Mulliken J.B., Glowacki J.: Classification of pediatric vascular lesions. *Plast. Reconstr. Surg.,* 1982; 70: 120-121.

Müssig K., Oksüz M.O., Pfannenberg C., Adam P., Zustin J., Beckert S., Petersenn S.: Somatostatin receptor expression in an epitheloid hemangioma causing oncogenic osteomalacia. *J. Clin. Endocrinol. Metab.,* 2009; 94: 4123-4124.

Ngan B.Y., Forte V., Campisi P.: Molecular angiogenic signaling in angiofibromas after embolization: implications for therapy. *Arch. Otolaryngol. Head Neck Surg.,* 2008; 134: 1170-1176.

Nguyen Q.D., De Wever O., Bruyneel E., Hendrix A., Xie W.Z., Lombet A., Leibl M., Mareel M., Gieseler F., Bracke M., Gespach C.: Commutators of PAR-1 signaling in cancer cell invasion reveal an essential role of the Rho-Rho kinase axis and tumor microenvironment. *Oncogene,* 2005; 24: 8240-8251.

Nicolai P., Schreiber A., Bolzoni Villaret A.: Juvenile angiofibroma: evolution of management. *Int. J. Pediatr.*, 2012; 2012: 412545.

Nikiforov Y.E., Seethala R.R., Tallini G., Baloch Z.W., Basolo F., Thompson L.D., Barletta J.A., Wenig B.M., Al Ghuzlan A., Kakudo K., Giordano T.J., Alves V.A., Khanafshar E., Asa S.L., El-Naggar A.K., Gooding W.E., Hodak S.P., Lloyd R.V., Maytal G., Mete O., Nikiforova M.N., Nosé V., Papotti M., Poller D.N., Sadow P.M., Tischler A.S., Tuttle R.M., Wall K.B., LiVolsi V.A., Randolph G.W., Ghossein R.A. Nomenclature Revision for Encapsulated Follicular Variant of Papillary Thyroid Carcinoma: A Paradigm Shift to Reduce Overtreatment of Indolent Tumors. *JAMA Oncol.* 2016; 2(8):1023-9.

Nonogaki S., Campos H.G., Butugan O., Soares F.A., Mangone F.R., Torloni H., Brentani M.M.: Markers of vascular differentiation, proliferation and tissue remodeling in juvenile nasopharyngeal angiofibromas. *Exp. Ther. Med.*, 2010; 1: 921-926.

Nozaki M., Sakurai E., Raisler B.J., Baffi J.Z., Witta J., Ogura Y., Brekken R.A., Sage E.H., Ambati B.K., Ambati J.: Loss of SPARC-mediated VEGFR-1 suppression after injury reveals a novel antiangiogenic activity of VEGF-A. *J. Clin. Invest.*, 2006; 116: 422-429.

Oates J, Clark J.R., Read J., Reeves N., Gao K., O'Brien C.J. Integration of prospective quality of life and nutritional assessment as routine components of multidisciplinary care of patients with head and neck cancer. *ANZ J Surg.* 2008 Jan-Feb; 78(1-2):34-41

Paran D., Elkayam O., Mayo A., Paran H., Amit M., Yaron M., Caspi D.: A pilot study of a long acting somatostatin analogue for the treatment of refractory rheumatoid arthritis. *Ann. Rheum. Dis.*, 2001; 60: 888-891.

Parker B.S., Argani P., Cook B.P., Liangfeng H., Chartrand S.D., Zhang M., Saha S., Bardelli A., Jiang Y., St. Martin T.B., Nacht M., Teicher B.A., Klinger K.W., Sukumar S., Madden S.L.: Alterations in vascular gene expression in invasive breast carcinoma. *Cancer Res.*, 2004; 64: 7857- 7866.

Pavlov K.A., Dubova E.A., Shchyogolev A.I., Mishnyov O.D.: Expression of growth factors in endotheliocytes in vascular malformations. *Bull. Exp. Biol. Med.,* 2009; 147: 366-370.

Pena I., Clayman G.L., Grubbs E.G., Bergeron J.M. Jr., Waguespack S.G., Cabanillas M.E., Dadu R., Hu M.I., Fellman B.M., Li Y., Gross N.D., Lai S.Y., Sturgis E.M., Zafereo M.E. Management of the lateral neck compartment in patients with sporadic medullary thyroid cancer. *Head Neck.* 2018; 40(1):79-85.

Pereira R., Quang C.T., Lesault I., Dolznig H., Beug H., Ghysdael J.: FLI-1 inhibits differentiation and induces proliferation of primary erythroblasts. *Oncogene,* 1999; 18: 1597-1608.

Podhajcer O.L., Benedetti L.G., Girotti M.R., Prada F., Salvatierra E., Llera A.S.: The role of the matricellular protein SPARC in the dynamic interaction between the tumor and the host. *Cancer Metastasis Rev.,* 2008; 27: 691-705.

Porter P.L., Sage E.H., Lane T.F., Funk S.E., Gown A.M.: Distribution of SPARC in normal and neoplastic human tissue. *J. Histochem. Cytochem.,* 1995; 43: 791-800.

Prada F., Benedetti L.G., Bravo A.I., Alvarez M.J., Carbone C., Podhajcer O.L.: SPARC endogenous level, rather than fibroblast-produced SPARC or stroma reorganization induced by SPARC, is responsible for melanoma cell growth. *J. Invest. Dermatol.,* 2007; 127: 2618-2628.

Qaisi, M., Eid, I. Pediatric Head and Neck Malignancies. *Oral and Maxillofacial Surgery Clinics,* 2016; 28(1):11-9.

Renkonen S., Heikkilä P., Haglund C., Mäkitie A.A., Hagström J.: Tenascin-C, GLUT-1, and syndecan-2 expression in juvenile nasopharyngeal angiofibroma: correlations to vessel density and tumor stage. *Head Neck,* 2013; 35: 1036-1042.

Resteghini, C., Trama, A., Borgonovi, E., Hosni, H., Corrao, G., Orlandi, E., Calareso, G., De Cecco, L., Piazza, C., Mainardi, L., Licitra, L. Big Data in Head and Neck Cancer. *Curr Treat Options Oncol,* 2018, 19(12):62.

Reubi J.C., Schaer J.C., Waser B., Mengod G.: Expression and localization of somatostatin receptor SSTR1, SSTR2, and SSTR3 messenger RNAs in primary human tumors using in situ hybridization. *Cancer Res.,* 1994; 54: 3455-3459.

Ringash, J., Bernstein, L.J., Devins, G., Dunphy, C., Giuliani, M., Martino, R., McEwen, S. Head and Neck Cancer Survivor ship: Learning the Needs, Meeting the Needs. *Semin Radiat Oncol,* 2018, 28(1):64-74.

Rio M.C.: From a unique cell to metastasis is a long way to go: clues to stromelysin-3 participation. *Biochimie,* 2005; 87: 299-306.

Rosenblatt S., Bassuk J.A., Alpers C.E., Sage E.H., Timpl R., Preissner K.T.: Differential modulation of cell adhesion by interaction between adhesive and counter-adhesive proteins: characterization of the binding of vitronectin to osteonectin (BM40, SPARC). *Biochem. J.,* 1997; 324: 311-319.

Rumpler G., Becker B., Hafner C., McClelland M., Stolz W., Landthaler M., Schmitt R., Bosserhoff A., Vogt T.: Identification of differentially expressed genes in models of melanoma progression by cDNA array analysis: SPARC, MIF and a novel cathepsin protease characterize aggressive phenotypes. *Exp. Dermatol.,* 2003; 12: 761-771.

Sage E.H.: Regulation of interactions between cells and extracellular matrix: a command performance on several stages. *J. Clin. Invest.,* 2001; 107: 781-783.

Said N., Socha M.J., Olearczyk J.J., Elmarakby A.A., Imig J.D., Motamed K.: Normalization of the ovarian cancer microenvironment by SPARC. *Mol. Cancer Res.,* 2007; 5: 1015-1030.

Shi Q., Bao S., Maxwell J.A., Reese E.D., Friedman H.S., Bigner D.D., Wang X.F., Rich J.N.: Secreted protein acidic, rich in cysteine (SPARC), mediates cellular survival of gliomas through AKT activation. *J. Biol. Chem.,* 2004; 279: 52200-52209.

Sim, F., Leidner, R., Bell, R.B. Immunotherapy for Head and Neck Cancer. *Hematol Oncol Clin North Am,* 2019; 33(2):301-321.

Singh A, Singhavi H, Sathe P, Mair M, Qayyumi B, Shetty R, Bal M, Joshi P, Nair S, Chaturvedi P. The impact of peritumoral depapillation in cancers of the tongue. *Oral Surg Oral Med Oral Pathol Oral Radiol.* 2020 Apr; 129(4):369-376.

Sosa M.S., Girotti M.R., Salvatierra E., Prada F., de Olmo J.A., Gallango S.J., Albar J.P., Podhajcer O.L., Llera A.S.: Proteomic analysis identified N-cadherin, clusterin, and HSP27 as mediators of SPARC (secreted protein, acidic and rich in cysteines) activity in melanoma cells. *Proteomics,* 2007; 7: 4123-4134.

Sure U., Freman S., Bozinov O., Benes L., Siegel A.M., Bertalanffy H.: Biological activity of adult cavernous malformations: a study of 56 patients. *J. Neurosurg.,* 2005; 102: 342-347.

Taïeb D., Varoquaux A., Chen C.C., Pacak K. Current and future trends in the anatomical and functional imaging of head and neck paragangliomas. *Semin Nucl Med.* 2013; 43(6):462-73.

Thewes M., Worret W.I., Engst R., Ring J.: Stromelysin-3 (ST-3): immunohistochemical characterization of the matrix metalloproteinase (MMP)-11 in benign and malignant skin tumours and other skin disorders. *Clin. Exp. Dermatol.,* 1999; 24: 122-126.

Thompson, L.D.R., Franchi, A. New tumor entities in the 4th edition of the World Health Organization classification of head and necktumors: Nasalcavity, paranasalsınuses and skullbase. *Virchows Arch.* 2018; 472(3): 315-330.

Tirakotai W., Fremann S., Soerensen N., Roggendorf W., Siegel A.M., Mennel H.D., Zhu Y., Bertalanffy H., Sure U.: Biological activity of paediatric cerebral cavernomas: an immunohistochemical study of 28 patients. *Childs Nerv. Syst.,* 2006; 22: 685-691.

Tsujie M., Uneda S., Tsai H., Seon B.K.: Effective anti-angiogenic therapy of established tumors in mice by naked anti-human endoglin (CD105) antibody: differences in growth rate and therapeutic response between tumors growing at different sites. *Int. J. Oncol.,* 2006; 29: 1087-1094.

Vikkula M., Boon L.M., Mulliken J.B.: Molecular genetics of vascular malformations. *Matrix Biol.,* 2001; 20: 327-335.

Wang Y., Qi F., Gu J.: Endothelial cell culture of intramuscular venous malformation and its invasive behavior related to matrix metalloproteinase-9. *Plast. Reconstr. Surg.,* 2009; 123: 1419-1430.

Watkins G., Douglas-Jones A., Bryce R., Mansel R.E., Jiang W.G.: Increased levels of SPARC (osteonectin) in human breast cancer tissues and its association with clinical outcomes. *Prostaglandins Leukot. Essent. Fatty Acids,* 2005; 72: 267-272.

Watson D.K., Smyth F.E., Thompson D.M., Cheng J.Q., Testa J.R., Papas T.S., Seth A.: The ERGB/Fli-1 gene: isolation and characterization of a new member of the family of human ETS transcription factors. *Cell Growth Differ.,* 1992; 3: 705-713.

Wendler O., Schäfer R., Schick B.: Mast cells and T-lymphocytes in juvenile angiofibromas. *Eur. Arch. Otorhinolaryngol.,* 2007; 264: 769-775.

Wennerberg J, Kjellén E, Lybak S, Rydell R, Pero R. Biochemical modulation of chemotherapy and radiotherapy in head and neck cancer. *Anticancer Res.* 1993; 13(6B):2501-6.

Winter P.F., Lapke J., Winek R.: Subcutaneous cavernous hemangioma visualized on an indium-111-octreotide scan. *J. Nucl. Med.,* 1996; 37: 1516-1517.

Wolf C., Chenard M.P., Durand de Grossouvre P., Bellocq J.P., Chambon P., Basset P.: Breast-cancer-associated stromelysin-3 gene is expressed in basal cell carcinoma and during cutaneous wound healing. *J. Invest. Dermatol.,* 1992; 99: 870-872.

Yamashita K., Tanaka Y., Mimori K., Inoue H., Mori M.: Differential expression of MMP and uPA systems and prognostic relevance of their expression in esophageal squamous cell carcinoma. *Int. J. Cancer,* 2004; 110: 201-207.

Yang E., Kang H.J., Koh K.H., Rhee H., Kim N.K., Kim H.: Frequent inactivation of SPARC by promoter hypermethylation in colon cancers. *Int. J. Cancer,* 2007; 121: 567-575.

Yi H., Fujimura Y., Ouchida M., Prasad D.D., Rao V.N., Reddy E.S.: Inhibition of apoptosis by normal and aberrant Fli-1 and erg proteins involved in human solid tumors and leukemias. *Oncogene,* 1997; 14: 1259-1268.

Yu Y., Fuhr J., Boye E., Gyorffy S., Soker S., Atala A., Mulliken J.B., Bischoff J.: Mesenchymal stem cells and adipogenesis in hemangioma involution. *Stem Cells,* 2006; 24: 1605-1612.

Zhang L., Eddy A., Teng Y.T., Fritzler M., Kluppel M., Melet F., Bernstein A.: An immunological renal disease in transgenic mice that overexpress Fli-1, a member of the ets family of transcription factor genes. *Mol. Cell. Biol.,* 1995; 15: 6961-6970.

Zhang M., Sun X., Yu H., Hu L., Wang D.: Biological distinctions between juvenile nasopharyngeal angiofibroma and vascular malformation: an immunohistochemical study. *Acta Histochem.,* 2011; 113: 626-630.

Zhang W., Liu Y., Chen X., Bergmeier S.C.: Novel inhibitors of basal glucose transport as potential anticancer agents. *Bioorg. Med. Chem. Lett.,* 2010; 20: 2191-2194.

Zou Y., Xiao X., Li Y., Zhou T.: Somatostatin analogues inhibit cancer cell proliferation in an SSTR2-dependent manner via both cytostatic and cytotoxic pathways. *Oncol. Rep.,* 2009; 21: 379-386.

In: A Biochemical View of Head and Neck ... ISBN: 978-1-53619-370-1
Editors: D. Bartusik-Aebisher et al. © 2021 Nova Science Publishers, Inc.

Chapter 3

BIOCHEMICAL STUDIES OF HEAD AND NECK CANCER TREATMENTS

*Lidia Bieniasz, David Aebisher, Wojciech Domka and Dorota Bartusik-Aebisher**
Medical College of The University of Rzeszów

ABSTRACT

Head and neck squamous cell carcinoma is an aggressive malignancy with high morbidity and mortality. Initial cancer assessment includes assessment of the histological appearance, tumor grading, lymph nodes status, and the presence of metastases. However, traditional diagnostic methods such as histopathology and radiology are not sensitive enough to detect a small number of neoplastic cells and are limited in their ability to predict treatment response. Recently, there has been significant progress in molecular diagnostics in these areas.

Keywords: head cancer, neck cancer, treatments

---

* Corresponding Author's Email: dbartusik-aebisher@ur.edu.pl.

Classical diagnostic methods, such as radiology and histopathology, have a limited sensitivity and only minimal residual disease can be detected with molecular techniques. Recent advancements in high-resolution imaging have improved the diagnostic assessment of magnetic resonance imaging (MRI) for intralabyrinthine schwannoma. This systematic review aimed to evaluate the diagnostic performance of MRI for patients. Only tumor-specific markers can be used in tissue samples containing normal tumor tissue counterpart, while in other samples, tissue-specific markers can be used. Neoplasms of the head and neck region are diagnosed in Poland in approximately 11,000 people annually. Over the last ten years, the number of cancer patients in this group has increased by as much as 25%. Neoplasms in the head and neck regions include:

- lip tumors
- oral cancer
- cancers of the mouth, larynx, nasopharynx
- laryngeal tumors
- salivary gland tumors
- nasal sinus tumors
- nasal cavity cancer
- Hearing cancer (ear cancer)

Squamous cell carcinomas account for 90% of head and neck cancers. The most common cancer of this localization is laryngeal cancer.

There are currently two main methodologies in use, one based on antigen-antibody interactions and the other based on amplified nucleic acids. The most commonly used nucleic acid markers are mutations or changes in tumor DNA or mRNA with different expression. Numerous reports and reviews have been published on the evaluation of minimal residual disease with molecular markers showing positive or negative clinical correlations. Here, we review recent studies evaluating performance in head and neck cancer care, from those spanning all phases of head and neck cancer. MR-guided radiotherapy requires novel quality assurance methods for intensity-modulated radiotherapy treatment plans

Here, an optimized method for TPs for a 1.5 T MR-linac was developed and implemented clinically. A static solid phantom and an MR-compatible 2D ionization chamber array were used.

Diagnostics in these tumors include:

- interview,
- medical examination with the assessment of the cervical and supraclavicular lymph nodes,
- ENT examination, including endoscopic examination (viewing with a flexible speculum of the larynx and its surroundings),
- biopsy of suspicious lesions (surgical removal of a sample from suspicious places or their puncture with a thin needle),
- imaging tests (including computed tomography or magnetic resonance imaging),
- ultrasound of the neck lymph nodes.

These tests are necessary to accurately determine the stage of clinical advancement.

In 2007 American Head and Neck Society expanded strategies to improve the quality of head and neck cancer care. In addition to underscoring the need for better training, multidisciplinary and regionalized care, and increased promotion of and adherence to clinical practice guidelines, he emphasized the need for developing quality metrics to measure, benchmark, and monitor the quality of head and neck cancer care. The development and maintenance of such indicators and metrics are now being required by federal regulations as markers of physician and institutional performance (Lewis et al., 2018).

The diagnostics for neck and cancer tumor is:

Esophagoscopy involves inserting a camera into the esophagus and allowing the mucosa to be viewed and samples to be taken for histopathological (microscopic) examination.

- Radiological examination of the upper gastrointestinal tract using contrast means taking a series of x-rays while the contrast is passing through the esophagus
- Bronchofiberoscopy - endoscopic examination of the airways for tumors in the middle or upper esophagus. It allows to identify possible infiltration of the respiratory system
- Computed tomography - a standard examination performed in patients who are to be qualified for surgery or radiotherapy.
- Positron emission computed tomography allows for a more accurate assessment of the stage of the disease.

Magnetic resonance Imaging allows for to localize the tumor.

The severity of the disease is of major importance for the effectiveness of treatment and the chances of a cure. The choice of therapy should be determined at a consensus by an interdisciplinary team of specialists. The following should be taken into account: detailed tumor location, histopathological result, clinical stage and patient's age.

In the first and second degree, the therapy is adapted to the location of the cancer, depending on the type of cancer - the applications are surgery, radiotherapy and brachytherapy.

Advanced stages of the disease - stage III and IV - require combined treatment. First of all, surgical treatment is used, the aim of which is to completely excise the tumor together with a part of healthy tissue. Additionally, when it is uncertain as to the completeness of the procedure, radiotherapy or radiochemotherapy is used.

Some patients with recurrent or generalized squamous cell carcinoma of the head and neck may receive immunotherapy (as part of a drug program). Treatment outcomes are also improved by the use of molecular targeted therapy (cetuximab).

The application of proton beam radiation therapy in the treatment of head and neck cancer has grown tremendously in the past few years. Globally, widespread interest in proton beam therapy has led to multiple research efforts regarding its therapeutic value and cost-effectiveness. The current standard of care using modern photon radiation technology has demonstrated excellent treatment outcomes, yet there are some situations where disease control remains suboptimal with the potential for detrimental acute and chronic toxicities. The proton beam, proton beam therapy may be superior to photon therapy in some patient subsets for both disease control and patient quality of life (Kim et al., 2018). Electrochemotherapy, the combination of electroporation and chemotherapy, is mainly used in the palliative setting for treatment of cutaneous and subcutaneous metastases. In the setting of local recurrence with no further curative treatment options available, electrochemotherapy could be of value. Scientist therefore performed a systematic search of the present literature. Eligible studies presented data from patients with head and neck cancer treated across the mucosal surface with electrochemotherapy. Overall complete response was reported as good, especially in primary small tumors. Side effects were minor in primary tumors whereas large, recurrent tumors displayed more frequent side effects and some serious adverse events. Design and structure of the studies differed considerably, making general comparisons difficult. Few studies concerning electrochemotherapy on mucosal head and neck tumors are available (Plaschke et al., 2016). The most common type of head and neck tumors are squamous cell cancer of the pharynx, the oral cavity and the larynx. These tumors can be treated by primary radio (chemo)therapy or surgery as well as a combination of both modalities depending on the site and extent of disease. This article will outline the recent developments in radiation therapy and give an overview of the potential long-term sequelae and their influencing factors (Schoch et al., 2016). Immunohistochemistry is a useful tool for diagnosing salivary gland and head and neck tumors. To review immunohistochemical markers, which can aid in the diagnosis of selected salivary gland and head and neck tumors. Salivary gland and head and neck tumors include a large diverse group of tumors with complex and overlapping histologic features. Immunohistochemistry plays an important role in resolving the differential diagnosis of some salivary gland and head and neck tumors and can provide information for the prognosis of certain tumors (Zhu et al., 2015). To quantify intrafractional motion to determine population-based radiotherapy treatment margins for head-and-neck tumors. Cine MR imaging was performed in 100 patients with head-and-neck cancer on a 3T scanner in a radiotherapy treatment setup. MR images were analyzed using deformable image registration and changes in tumor contour position were used to calculate the tumor motion. The tumor motion was used together with patient setup errors to calculate population-based margins (Bruijnen et al., 2019). Although the average tumor motion was small, tumor motion varied considerably between patients (0.1-12.0 mm). Desmoid tumors often grow locally, invasively, and may, in rare instances, be fatal secondary to invasion into critical structures, such as airway or major vessels. The most common treatment is surgery, but desmoid tumors are characteristically associated with a high local recurrence rate after resection (de Bree et al., 2013). External beam radiation therapy is a commonly utilized treatment modality in the management of head and neck cancer. Given the close proximity of disease to critical normal tissues and structures, the delivery of external beam radiation therapy can result in severe acute and late toxicities, even when delivered with advanced photon-based techniques, such as intensity-modulated radiation therapy (Ahn et al., 2014). Proton beam radiation has been used for cancer treatment since the 1950s, but recent increasing interest in this form of therapy and the construction of hospital-based and clinic-based facilities for its delivery have greatly increased both the number of patients and the variety of tumors being treated with proton therapy (Holliday et al., 2014). Radiation dose escalation and acceleration improves local control but also increases toxicity. Proton radiation is an emerging therapy for localized cancers that is being sought with increasing frequency by patients. Compared with photon therapy, proton therapy spares more critical structures due to its unique physics. The physical properties of a proton beam make it ideal for clinical applications (Liu et al., 2011). Head and neck cancer is a fatal malignancy with an overall long-term survival of about 50% for all stages. The diagnosis is not rarely delayed, and the majority of patients present with loco-regionally advanced disease (Guidi et al., 2018). Treatment of head and neck cancer with surgery and radiotherapy and sometimes combined with adjuvant chemotherapy depending on the tumor site, extent, and histology (Mendenhall et al., 2019). The head and neck region harbor numerous specialized tissues of all lineages giving rise to a plethora of different malignancies. In this overview, scientist present the most recent developments in the classification, histopathological characteristics, and molecular features of head and neck cancer (Andreasen et al., 2019). Head and neck squamous cell carcinoma is a frequent tumour arising from multiple anatomical subsites in the head and neck region (Rothschild et al., 2018). Improvement in outcomes are needed for patients with recurrent and or metastatic squamous cell carcinoma of the head and neck. In 2016, the US Food and Drug Administration granted inhibitors nivolumab and pembrolizumab - for the treatment of patients with recurrent squamous cell carcinoma of the head and neck (Cohen et al., 2019). In 2019, the FDA granted approval pembrolizumab in combination with platinum and fluorouracil for all patients with HNSCC and pembrolizumab as a single agent for patients with HNSCC whose tumors express a PD-L1 combined positive score ≥ 1 (Cohen et al., 2019).

For head and neck neoplasms, the clinical advancement classification of TNM applies. It determines the degree of tumor spread in the body through each feature.

Feature T - determines the size of the tumor, its location and spread inside normal tissues.

Feature N - determines the size of the lymph node metastasis and the number of lymph nodes involved.

Feature M - defines the existence of tumor metastases in tissues distant from the initial organ - the degree of tumor spread

Cancer immunotherapy has led this endeavour, attempting to improve tumour recognition and expand immune responses against tumour cells. This article will review biological mechanisms of immune escape and implications for immunotherapy in HNSCC (Moy et al., 2017). Radiotherapy is one of the key treatment modalities used in head and neck cancer management. This paper summarises the current role and some of the recent advances in radiotherapy in head and neck cancer management (Nutting, 2016). Typically head and neck cancer patients will have radiation therapy which is based on the state-of-the-art imaging technology including computed tomography, magnetic resonance imaging, positron emission tomography or other imaging techniques. Concomitant and alternating chemoradiotherapy treatments are also acceptable in larynx preservation (Denaro et al., 2014). Xerostomia is the most common late side-effect of radiotherapy to the head and neck. Compared with conventional radiotherapy, intensity-modulated radiotherapy can reduce irradiation of the parotid glands (Nutting et al., 2011). Radiomics is aimed at image-based tumor phenotyping, enabling application within clinical-decision-support-systems to improve diagnostic accuracy and allow for personalized treatment. The purpose was to identify predictive 18-fluor-fluoro-2-deoxyglucose (^{18}F-FDG) positron-emission tomography (PET) radiomic features to predict recurrence, distant metastasis, and overall survival in patients with head and neck squamous cell carcinoma treated with chemoradiotherapy. This randomized trial compared the rates of delayed xerostomia between two-dimensional radiation therapy and intensity-modulated radiation therapy in the treatment of early-stage nasopharyngeal carcinoma (Kam et al., 2007). Our previous individual patient data meta-analysis showed that chemotherapy improved survival in patients curatively treated for non-metastatic head and neck squamous cell carcinoma, with a higher benefit with concomitant chemotherapy. The log-rank-test, stratified by trial, was used to compare treatments. The hazard ratios of death were calculated (Pignon et al., 2009). The recently updated meta-analysis of chemotherapy in head and neck cancer demonstrated the benefit of the addition of chemotherapy in terms of overall survival in head and neck squamous cell carcinoma (Blanchard et al., 2011). The primary end point was the duration of control of locoregional disease; secondary end points were overall survival, progression-free survival, the response rate, and safety (Bonner et al., 2006; Bernier et al., 2004). Patients with squamous-cell carcinoma of the head and neck who received docetaxel plus cisplatin and fluorouracil induction chemotherapy plus chemoradiotherapy had a significantly longer survival than did patients who received cisplatin and fluorouracil induction chemotherapy plus chemoradiotherapy (Posner et al., 2007). As compared with the standard regimen of cisplatin and fluorouracil, induction chemotherapy with the addition of docetaxel significantly improved progression-free and overall survival in patients with unresectable squamous-cell carcinoma of the head and neck (Vermorken et al., 2007). Chemotherapy plays a definite role in the management of head and neck cancers, especially in combination with radiotherapy in patients with possibly curable disease (Devriendt, et al., 1997). The immune system plays a key role in the development, establishment, and progression of head and neck squamous cell carcinoma. Through the tumor's influence on the microenvironment, the immune system can be exploited to promote metastasis, angiogenesis, and growth (Devriendt, et al., 1997). Magnetic resonance imaging performed in cancer diagnostics is extremely accurate and enables the observation of our internal organs in all planes. For this reason, it has a significant advantage over both ultrasound and computed tomography, and is ideal, especially in the case of imaging those tissues in which tumors develop most often. However, what are the main indications for an MRI scan? In oncological diagnostics, MRI is performed to detect tumors of the lungs, brain, pancreas, liver, stomach, bladder, kidneys, thyroid gland, and genital organs. Due to the fact that the MRI is painless and non-invasive, it can be performed many times. In order to obtain a more precise image of our body, the so-called contrast, which is a special substance administered intravenously, which accumulates inside our tissues, helps to strengthen the above-mentioned signal. Unfortunately, not every person can be tested with contrast, because this substance should not be used by people with renal insufficiency, as well as women during pregnancy. Immune system dysfunction plays a role in both the development and progression of head and neck squamous cell carcinoma, highlighting the potential role for immunotherapy to improve outcomes in this disease (Ling et al., 2018). Morbidity and quality of life issues are major challenges in this patient population due to the debilitating effects of standard of care treatment paradigms. There is a critical need for new therapeutic approaches to manage HNSCC with better anti-tumor activities and toxicity profiles. Immunotherapy has gained traction as a precision medicine initiative to manage solid malignancies (Xie, et al., 2017). Evidence to date shows that immune checkpoint inhibitors have little benefit in most patients with head and neck squamous cell carcinoma. Intense interest is focused on identifying and developing rational combinations of immune checkpoint inhibitors and different therapeutic interventions to enhance response rates and overcome immune checkpoint inhibitor resistance (Karam et al., 2019). The immune system has a vital role in the development, establishment, and progression of head and neck squamous cell carcinoma. Immune evasion of cancer cells leads to progression of HNSCC. An understanding of this mechanism provides the basis for improved therapies and outcomes for patients. Through the tumor's influence on the microenvironment, the immune system can be exploited to promote metastasis, angiogenesis, and growth (Sim et al., 2019). MR-guided radiotherapy requires novel quality assurance methods for intensity-modulated radiotherapy treatment plans Here, an optimized method for TPs for a 1.5 T MR-linac was developed and implemented clinically. A static solid phantom and an MR-compatible 2D ionization chamber array were used. Head and neck squamous cell carcinomas arise in the mucosal linings of the upper aerodigestive tract and are unexpectedly heterogeneous in nature. In 2015, The Cancer Genome Atlas consortium published a comprehensive molecular catalogue on HNSCC. In 2016, the first results of immunotherapy trials with immune checkpoint inhibitors were published, and these may be considered as a paradigm shift in head and neck oncology (Leemans et al., 2018). Patients with advanced head and neck cancers who are not eligible for curative treatment represent a challenging cohort of patients to manage given the complexity and severity of their presenting symptoms. Palliative radiation therapy, along with other systemic and surgical measures, has the potential to significantly improve the quality of life of such patients. There is little high-level evidence and a lack of consensus to direct the selection of an optimal palliative radiation regimen. An ideal palliative radiation regimen should alleviate symptoms secondary to the cancer with minimal treatment toxicity and side effects while improving a patient's quality of life. This review presents the treatment approaches, outcomes, and toxicities associated with different radiation regimens and proposes a multidisciplinary framework for the selection of an individualized treatment regimen for patients that centers around patient prognosis, goals of care, logistics of treatment, and the availability of other surgical and systemic therapies (Grewal et al., 2019; Iqbal et al., 2018). The objective of this systematic review was to identify and appraise the existing evidence of role of palliative radiotherapy for locally advanced non-metastatic head and neck cancer (Zackrisson et al., 2003). There is a non-significant trend for the overall survival being lower in non-surgically treated patients than in those treated with primary surgery and postoperative radiotherapy (Blanchard et al., 2019). Cancer of the head and neck is a heterogeneous disease of the upper aerodigestive tract, encompassing distinct histologic types, different anatomic sites, and human papillomaviruspositive as well as HPV-negative cancers. Advanced/recurrent HNCs have poor prognosis with low survival rates. Tumor-mediated inhibition of antitumor immune responses and a high mutational burden are common features of HNCs. Both are responsible for the successful escape of these tumors from the host immune system. Dysfunctional immune cells in patients with recurrent/metastatic HNC can be made effective by the delivery of immunotherapies in combination with conventional treatments (Whiteside, 2018).

CONCLUSION

Efficiency of immune therapies is expected to rapidly improve with the possibility for patients' selection based on personal immunogenomic profiles. Noninvasive biomarkers of response to therapy will be emerging as a better understanding of the various molecular signals co-opted by the tumors is gained.

REFERENCES

Ahmad, P; Sana, J; Slavik, M; Slampa, P; Smilek, P; Slaby, O. Micro RNAs Involvement in Radio resistance of Head and Neck Cancer. *DisMarkers*, 2017.

Ahn, PH; Lukens, JN; Boon-Keng, KT; Kirk, M; Lin, A. The use of proton therapy in the treatment of head and neckcancers. *Cancer J*, 2014, 20(6), 421-6.

Atkins, Jr. JP; Keane, WM; Young, KA; Rowe, LD. Value of panendoscopy in determination of second primary cancer. A study of 451 cases of head and neck cancer. *Arch Otolaryngol*, 1984, 110(8), 533-4.

Bernier, J; Domenge, C; Ozsahin, M; Matuszewska, K; Lefèbvre, JL; Greiner, RH; et al. Postoperative irradiation with or without concomitant chemotherapy for locally advanced head and neck cancer. *N Engl J Med*, 2004, 350(19), 1945-52.

Blanchard, P; Baujat, B; Holostenco, V; Bourredjem, A; Baey, C; Bourhis, J; et al. Meta-analysis of chemotherapy in head and neck cancer (MACH-NC): a comprehensive analysis by tumour site. *Radiother Oncol*, 2011, 100(1), 33-40.

Blanchard, P; Biau, J; Castelli, J; Tao, Y; Graff, P; Nguyen, F. [Individualization of dose and fractionation of radiotherapy for head and neck cancers]. *Cancer Radiother*, 2019, 23(6-7), 784-788.

Bonner, JA; Harari, PM; Giralt, J; Azarnia, N; Shin, DM; Cohen, RB; et al. Radiotherapy plus cetuximab for squamous-cell carcinoma of the head and neck. *N Engl J Med*, 2006, 354(6), 567-78.

Boppana, NB; Stochaj, U; Kodiha, M; Bielawska, A; Bielawski, J; Pierce, JS; Korbelik, M; Separovic, D. C6-pyridinium ceramide sensitizes SCC17B human head and neck squamous cell carcinoma cells to photodynamic therapy. *J Photochem Photobiol B*, 2015, 143, 163-8.

Bruijnen, T; Stemkens, B; Terhaard, CHJ; Lagendijk, JJW; Raaijmakers, CPJ; Tijssen, RHN. Intrafraction motion quantification and planning target volume margin determination of head-and-neck tumors using cine magnetic resonance imaging. *Radiotherapy & Oncology*, 2019, 130, 82-88.

Caudell, JJ; Torres-Roca, JF; Gillies, RJ; Enderling, H; Kim, S; Rishi, A; Moros, EG; Harrison, LB. The future of personalized radiotherapy for head and neckcancer. *Lancet Oncol*, 2017.

Chen, WH; Lecarosb, RLG; Tsengc, YC; Huangc, L; Hsud, YC. Nanoparticle delivery of HIF1α siRNA combined with photodynamic therapy as a potential treatment strategy for head-and-neck cancer, *CancerLett.*, 2015, 359(1), 65-74.

Chloupek, A; Zarzycki, K; Dąbrowski, J; Domański, W. Parotidgland tumors. Results of retrospective analysis of 149 patients treated at the Clinical Department of Cranio-Maxillofacial Surgery, Clinic of Otolaryngology and Oncologic Laryngology of Military Institute of Medicine in Warsaw in years 2006-2016. *Otolaryngol Pol*, 2017.

Cohen, EEW; Bell, RB; Bifulco, CB; Burtness, B; Gillison, ML; Harrington, KJ; Le, QT; Lee, NY; Leidner, R; Lewis, RL; Licitra, L; Mehanna, H; Mell, LK; Raben, A; Sikora, AG; Uppaluri, R; Whitworth, F; Zandberg, DP; Ferris, RL. The Society for Immunotherapy of Cancer consensus statement on immunotherapy for the treatment of squamous cell carcinoma of the head and neck (HNSCC). *J Immunother Cancer*, 2019, 7(1), 184.

de Bree, E; Zoras, O; Hunt, JL; Takes, RP; Suárez, C; Mendenhall, WM; Hinni, ML. Desmoid tumors of the head and neck: A therapeutic challenge. *Clinical Review*, 2014, 36(10), 1517-26.

Denaro, N; Russi, EG; Lefebvre, JL; Merlano, MC. A systematic review of current and emerging approaches in the field of larynx preservation. *Radiother Oncol*, 2014, 110(1), 16-24.

Devriendt, D; Klastersky, J. New cytostatic agents for the treatment of head and neck cancer. *Acta Otorhinolaryngol Belg*, 1997, 51(2), 61-8.

Ferris, RL. Immunology and Immunotherapy of Head and Neck Cancer. *J Clin Oncol*, 2015, 33(29), 3293–3304.

Grewal, AS; Jones, J; Lin, A. Palliative Radiation Therapy for Head and Neck Cancers. *Int J Radiat Oncol Biol Phys*, 2019, 105(2), 254-266.

Guidi, A; Codecà, C; Ferrari, D. Chemotherapy and immunotherapy for recurrent and metastatic head and neck cancer: a systematic review. *Med Oncol*, 2018, 35(3), 37.

He, C; Liu, D; Lin, W. Self-assembled core-shell nanoparticles for combined chemotherapy and photodynamic therapy of resistant head and neck cancers. *ACS Nano*, 2015.

Holliday, EB; Frank, ST. Proton radiation therapy for head and neck cancer: a review of the clinical experience to date. *Int J Radiat Oncol Biol Phys*, 2014, 89(2), 292-302.

Kaidar-Person, O; Gil, Z; Billan, S. Precision medicine in head and neck cancer, *Drug Resist Updat*, 2018.

Kam, MK; Leung, SF; Zee, B; Chau, RM; Suen, JJ; Mo, F; et al. Prospective randomized study of intensity-modulated radiotherapy on salivary gland function in early-stage nasopharyngeal carcinoma patients. *J Clin Oncol*, 2007, 25(31), 4873-9.

Karam, SD; Raben, D. Radio immunotherapy for the treatment of head and neck cancer. *Lancet Oncol*, 2019, 20, e404–16.

Katabi, N; Lewis, JS. Update from the 4th Edition of the World Health Organization Classification of Head and Neck Tumours: What Is New in the 2017 WHO Blue Book for Tumors and Tumor-Like Lesions of the Neck and Lymph Nodes. *Head Neck Pathol*, 2017 Mar, 11(1), 48-54.

Kim, JK; Leeman, JE; Riaz, N; McBride, S; Tsai, CJ; Lee, NY. Proton Therapy for Head and Neck Cancer. *Curr Treat Options Oncol*, 2018, 19(6), 28.

Kiss, SAK; Mikkelsen, LH; Channir, HI; Plaschke, CC; Melchior, LC; Eriksen, JG; Wessel, I. An update on head and neck cancer: new entities and their histopathology, molecular back ground, treatment, and out come. *APMIS*, 2019, 127, 240–264.

Lee, SJ; Hwang, HJ; Shin, JI; Ahn, JC; Chung, PS. Enhancement of cytotoxic effect on human head and neck cancer cells by combination of photodynamic therapy and sulforaphane. *Gen Physiol Biophys*, 2015, 34(1), 13-21.

Leemans, CR; Snijders, PJF; Brakenhoff, RH. The molecular landscape of head and neck cancer. *Nat Rev Cancer*, 2018, 18(5), 269-282.

Ling, DC; Bakkenist, CJ; Ferris, RL; Clump, DA. Role of Immunotherapy in Head and Neck Cancer. *Semin Radiat Oncol*, 2018, 28(1), 12-16.

Liu, H; Joe, Y. Chang. Proton therapy in clinical practice. *Chin J Cancer*, 2011, 30(5), 315-26.

Lu, K; He, C; Lin, W. Nanoscale Metal–Organic Framework for Highly Effective Photodynamic Therapy of Resistant Head and Neck Cancer. *J Am Chem Soc.*, 2014, 9(1), 991-1003.

Marchal, S; Dolivet, G; Lassalle, HP; Guillemin, F; Bezdetnaya, L. Targeted photodynamic therapy in head and neck squamous cell carcinoma: heading into the future. *Lasers in Medical Science*, 2015, 30(9), 2381-2387.

Mendenhall, WM; Dagan, R; Bryant, CM; Fernandes, RP. Radiation Oncology for Head and Neck Cancer: Current Standards and Future Changes. *Oral Maxillofac Surg Clin North Am*, 2019, 31(1), 31-38.

Moy, JD; Moskovitz, JM; Ferris, RL. Biological mechanisms of immune escape and implications for immunotherapy in head and neck squamous cell carcinoma. *Eur J Cancer*, 2017, 76, 152-166.

Nutting, CM; Morden, JP; Harrington, KJ; Urbano, TG; Bhide, SA; Clark, C; et al. Parotid-sparing intensity modulated versus conventional radiotherapy in head and neck cancer (PARSPORT): a phase 3 multicentre randomised controlled trial. *Lancet Oncol*, 2011, 12(2), 127-36.

Nutting, C. Radiotherapy in head and neck cancer management: United Kingdom National Multidisciplinary Guidelines. *The Journal of Laryngology & Otology*, 2016, 130(Suppl 2), S66–S67.

Pignon, JP; Maitre, A; Maillard, E; Bourhi, J. Group M-NC. Meta-analysis of chemotherapy in head and neck cancer (MACH-NC), an update on 93 randomised trials and 17,346 patients. *Radiother Oncol*, 2009, 92(1), 4-14.

Posner, MR; Hershock, DM; Blajman, CR; Mickiewicz, E; Winquist, E; Gorbounova, V; et al. Cisplatin and fluorouracil alone or with docetaxel in head and neck cancer. *N Engl J Med*, 2007, 357(17), 1705-15.

Qaisi, M; Eid, I. Pediatric Head and Neck Malignancies. *Oral and Maxillofacial Surgery Clinics*, 2016-02-01, Volume 28, Issue 1, Pages 11-19, Copyright © 2016 Elsevier Inc.

Resteghini, C; Trama, A; Borgonovi, E; Hosni, H; Corrao, G; Orlandi, E; Calareso, G; De Cecco, L; Piazza, C; Mainardi, L; Licitra, L. Big Data in Head and Neck Cancer. *Curr Treat Options Oncol*, 2018.

Ringash, J; Bernstein, LJ; Devins, G; Dunphy, C; Giuliani, M; Martino, R; McEwen, S. Head and Neck Cancer Survivorship: Learning the Needs, Meeting the Needs. *Semin Radiat Oncol*, 2018.

Rothschild, U; Muller, L; Lechner, A; Schlösser, HA; Beutner, D; Läubli, H; Zippelius, A; Rothschild, SI. Immunotherapy in head and neck cancer – scientific rationale, current treatment options and future directions. *Swiss Med Wkly*, 2018, 2018, 148, w14625.

Schoch, M; Däppen, MB; Henke, G; Stöckli, S. Long-term sequelae after chemo radiation in head neck tumors. *Ther Umsch.*, 2016, 73(4), 213-8.

ShahidIqbal, M; Kelly, C; Kovarik, J; Goranov, B; Shaikh, G; Morgan, D; Dobrowsky, W; Paleri, V. Palliative radiotherapy for locally advanced non-metastatic head and neck cancer: A systematic review. *Radiother Oncol*, 2018, 126(3), 558-567.

Sim, F; Leidner, R; Bell, RB. Immunotherapy for Head and Neck Cancer. *Oral Maxillofac Surg Clin North Am*, 2019, 31(1), 85-100.

Sim, F; Leidner, R; Bell, RB. Immunotherapy for Head and Neck Cancer. *Hematol Oncol Clin North Am*, 2019.

Thompson, LDR; Franchi, A. *New tumor entities in the 4th edition of the World Health Organization classification of head and necktumors: Nasalcavity, paranasalsinuses and skullbase. Virchows Arch.*, 2018 Mar, 472(3), 315-330.

Vermorken, JB; Remenar, E; van Herpen, C; Gorlia, T; Mesia, R; Degardin, M; et al. Cisplatin, fluorouracil, and docetaxel in unresectable head and neck cancer. *N Engl J Med*, 2007, 357(17), 1695-704.

Whiteside, TL. Head and Neck Carcinoma Immunotherapy: Facts and Hopes. *Clin Cancer Res*, 2018, 24(1), 6-13.

Wojdas, W; Kosek, J; Dżaman, K; Szczygielski, K; Ratajczak, J; Jurkiewicz, D. Zastosowanie laserów w leczeniu chorób krtani

[Application of lasers in treatment of larynx diseases]. *Otolaryngol Pol*, 2009, 63 (7), 76-79.

Xie, X; O'Neill, W; Pan, Q. Immunotherapy for head and neck cancer: the future of treatment? *Expert Opin Biol Ther*, 2017, 17(6), 701-708.

Zackrisson, B; Mercke, C; Strander, H; Wennerberg, J; Cavallin-Ståhl, E. A systematic overview of radiation therapy effects in head and neck cancer. *Acta Oncol, 2003*, 42(5-6), 443-61.

Zhu, S; Schuerch, C Hunt, J. Review and updates of immunohistochemistry in selected salivary gland and head and necktumors. *Arch Pathol Lab Med.*, 2015 Jan, 139(1), 55-66.

Chapter 4

BIOCHEMICAL STUDIES OF HEAD AND NECK CANCER BIOMARKERS

Wojciech Domka, David Aebisher, Lidia Bieniasz and Dorota Bartusik-Aebisher*
Medical College of The University of Rzeszów, Poland

ABSTRACT

Cancer cells represent a specific metabolic state. Targeted therapies are urgently needed in order to minimize the treatment toxicity.

Keywords: head, neck, cancer, markers

Head and neck cancers (including those of the lip and oral cavity, nasal cavity, paranasal sinuses, oropharynx, larynx and nasopharynx) represent nearly 700 000 new cases. There is 380,000 deaths worldwide per annum, and account for over 10,000 annual deaths in the United States alone (Moy et al., 2017). Tumor markers are substances that are selectively released by

---

* Corresponding Author's Email: dbartusik-aebisher@ur.edu.pl.

cancer cells into the bloodstream and can therefore be detected in serum or other body fluids for clinical monitoring.

Serum markers fall into three main categories:

- antigens
- carbohydrate antigens as part of glycolipids or glycolipoproteins
- miscellaneous, including tissue-specific enzymes. protein cytoskeleton

Most carbohydrate antigens that are useful in the diagnosis of human cancer exhibit tumor-specific abnormal glycosylation, with O instead of N linkage to protein residues. To date, not a single biomarker or panel of biomarkers for the detection of head and neck tumors has been detected that could be clinically used.

The limitations of the clinical use of the biomarkers are:

- primarily the heterogeneity of the studied groups
- the low sensitivity
- the low specificity of the biomarkers during the study (Gronkiewicz et al., 2014).

The mentioned markers are currently the subjects of multidirectional studies in oncology, as they take part in the process of neoangiogenesis and proliferation of tumors (Gronkiewicz et al., 2014). The problem of diagnosis in the field of head and neck region is still valid. Specificdiagnosis and precise estimation of the tumor's size with the use of CT and MRI imaging is generally unsatisfactory. The Positron Emission Tomography (PET) supports this process with additional information about the tumor's metabolism. Numerous publications show that PET-CT has a great influence on the evaluation of the size of the tumor, presence of lymph node metastases, choice of treatment and the prognosis of the recurrence.

These abnormalities might be used as the neoplastic markers (Czarnecka et al., 2009). Vascular anomalies are congenital errors in vascular development. Because treatment options for vascular anomalies are widely variable and often debated, this report aims to provide a comprehensive approach to these lesions based upon current concepts and practical clinical experience (Buckmiller et al., 2010). Radiotherapy is an integral component in the management of head and neck cancer. These challenges could potentially be addressed by means of personalized treatment (Andreassen et al., 2018). Preclinical data suggest that head and neck squamous cell carcinoma is a profoundly immunosuppressive disease, characterized by abnormal secretion of proinflammatory cytokines and dysfunction of immune effector cells (Gavrielatou et al., 2020). Historically, the term tumor marker refers to a biological or biochemical substance selectively released by tumor cells into the circulation, which can then be detected in blood serum or other body fluids for clinical monitoring of the tumor process.

Tumor markers are useful in all phases of the diagnostic process:

- Screening tests (cancer prevention).
- Recognition of an ongoing neoplastic process in correlation with specific symptoms.
- Determining the stage of disease advancement (dependence of the marker expression level on the advancement of the neoplastic process)
- Localization of neoplastic changes within the organ
- Monitoring the effectiveness of treatment (evaluation of disease progression / regression after surgery, radio- and chemotherapy, detection of recurrence)
- Setting a therapeutic target for new drugs

An ideal tumor marker is a substance which is not normally present in the circulation, the detection of which in the serum in even minimal amounts reflects the presence, progression or regression of an ongoing neoplastic process (Mlak et al., 2010). This method in comparison with radiotherapy alone produces significant benefit in overall survival. The most recognized and well investigated target of molecular treatment for

SCHNC is epidermal growth factor receptor (Kawecki et al., 2010). EGFR signaling pathway activation is associated with tumor progression and stimulation of chemo- and radioresistance (Magdelénat et al., 1992). Historically, tumour markers are substances selectively released by tumour cells in the blood stream so that they can be detected in the serum or other body fluids for clinical monitoring of various malignancies.

Validated prognostic, predictive, and toxicity markers should help cancer treatment move from the current trial-and-error approach to more personalized treatment (Duffy et al., 2010). Therefore, it is of great importance to develop diagnostic methods that allow for earlier detection of the disease, as well as a better assessment of its advancement and the choice of therapy. The evaluation of these markers in the treatment process and in the long-term follow-up of patients after treatment is more widely used (Soborczyk et al., 2007). In spite of a rapidly expanding understanding of head and neck tumor biology as well as optimization of radiation, chemotherapy, and surgical treatment modalities, head and neck squamous cell carcinoma remains a major cause of cancer related morbidity and mortality (Puram et al., 2015; Kemmer et al., 2018). Head and neck cancers encompass a heterogeneous group of tumours that, in general, are biologically aggressive in nature. These cancers remain difficult to treat and treatment can cause severe, long-term side effects. For patients who are not cured by surgery and/or (chemo)radiotherapy, there are few effective treatment options. This clinical update aims to provide an insight into the current understanding of the molecular pathogenesis of the disease, and explores the novel therapies under development and in clinical trials (Suh et al., 2014). The development and maintenance of such indicators and metrics are now being required by federal regulations as markers of physician and institutional performance (Lewis et al., 2018). The application of proton beam radiation therapy in the treatment of head and neck cancer has grown tremendously in the past few years. As enthusiasm and excitement for proton beam therapy continue to increase, clinical research and widespread adoption will elucidate the true value of proton beam therapy and give a greater understanding of the full risks and benefits of proton therapy in head and neck cancer (Kim et al., 2018).

Electrochemotherapy, the combination of electroporation and chemotherapy, is mainly used in the palliative setting for treatment of cutaneous and subcutaneous metastases; however, new applications are continuously being explored (Plaschke et al., 2016). Overall complete response was reported as good, especially in primary small tumors. Side effects were minor in primary tumors whereas large, recurrent tumors displayed more frequent side effects and some serious adverse events. Design and structure of the studies differed considerably, making general comparisons difficult. Few studies concerning electrochemotherapy on mucosal head and neck tumors are available and they are not easily comparable. Overall response to treatment is good; nonetheless, further systematic studies are warranted. The most common type of head and neck tumors are squamous cell cancer of the pharynx, the oral cavity and the larynx (Schoch et al., 2016). Context: Immunohistochemistry is a useful tool for diagnosing salivary gland and head and neck tumors. To review immunohistochemical markers, which can aid in the diagnosis of selected salivary gland and head and neck tumors (Zhu et al., 2015Bruijnen et al., 2019; Bruijnen et al., 2019). Desmoid tumor, or aggressive fibromatosis, is a rare, histologically benign, fibroblastic lesion that infrequently presents in the head and neck (de Bree et al., 2013). External beam radiation therapy is a commonly utilized treatment modality in the management of head and neck cancer. Ultimately, the widespread adaptation and implementation of proton therapy for head and neck cancer will require direct, prospective comparisons to standard techniques such as intensity-modulated radiation therapy, with a focus on measures such as toxicity, disease control, and quality of life (Ahn et al., 2014). Proton beam radiation has been used for cancer treatment since the 1950s, but recent increasing interest in this form of therapy and the construction of hospital-based and clinic-based facilities for its delivery have greatly increased both the number of patients and the variety of tumors being treated with proton therapy. multimodality therapy comprising surgery, radiation therapy, and chemotherapy. However, aggressive local therapy in the proximity of critical normal structures to tumors in the head and neck region may produce debilitating early and late toxic (Liu et al., 2011). Head and neck cancer is a fatal malignancy with an overall long-term survival of about 50% for all stages (Mendenhall et al., 2019). The prognosis is limited and novel treatment approaches are urgently needed (Rothschild et al., 2018). Radiotherapy is one of the key treatment modalities used in head and neck cancer management. Radiotherapy and surgery are the two most frequently used therapeutic modalities in head and neck cancer. For an advanced squamous cell carcinoma of the head and neck, single modality treatment is associated with poor outcomes. Typically head and neck cancer patients will have radiation therapy which is based on the state-of-the-art imaging technology including computed tomography, magnetic resonance imaging, positron emission tomography or other imaging techniques (Nutting et al., 2016). Treatment options targeting laryngeal preservation include conservative surgery, concurrent chemo-radiotherapy, induction chemotherapy followed by radiotherapy, and alternating chemo-radiation. Concomitant and alternating chemoradiotherapy treatments are also acceptable in larynx preservation (Denaro et al., 2014). Xerostomia is the most common late side-effect of radiotherapy to the head and neck. Compared with conventional radiotherapy, intensity-modulated radiotherapy can reduce irradiation of the parotid glands. (Nutting et al., 2011). The benefit of concomitant chemotherapy was confirmed and was greater than the benefit of induction chemotherapy. The recently updated meta-analysis of chemotherapy in head and neck cancer demonstrated the benefit of the addition of chemotherapy in terms of overall survival in head and neck squamous cell carcinoma (Blanchard et al., 2011). The scientist conducted a multinational, randomized study to compare radiotherapy alone with radiotherapy plus cetuximab, a monoclonal antibody against the epidermal growth factor receptor, in the treatment of locoregionally advanced squamous-cell carcinoma of the head and neck (Bonner et al., 2006). Treatment of locoregionally advanced head and neck cancer with concomitant high-dose radiotherapy plus cetuximab improves locoregional control and reduces mortality without increasing the common toxic effects associated with radiotherapy to the head and neck (Bernier et al., 2004). A randomized phase 3 trial of the treatment of squamous-cell carcinoma of the head and neck compared induction chemotherapy with docetaxel plus cisplatin and fluorouracil with cisplatin and fluorouracil, followed by chemoradiotherapy. Patients with squamous-cell carcinoma of the head and neck who received docetaxel plus cisplatin and fluorouracil induction chemotherapy plus chemoradiotherapy had a significantly longer survival than did patients who received cisplatin and fluorouracil induction chemotherapy plus chemoradiotherapy (Vermorken et al., 2007). As compared with the standard regimen of cisplatin and fluorouracil, induction chemotherapy with the addition of docetaxel significantly improved progression-free and overall survival in patients with unresectable squamous-cell carcinoma of the head and neck. Chemotherapy plays a definite role in the management of head and neck cancers, especially in combination with radiotherapy in patients with possibly curable disease. As far as new agents are concerned, the combinations of paclitaxel or docetaxel and gemcitabine with cisplatin or carboplatin deserve special attention. These regimens should be compared to the more classical combinations of cisplatin with 5efluorouracil or Ifosfamide in phase III trials. A special emphasis should be placed on the evaluation of these new agents in combination with radiotherapy, since all have strong radio potentiating properties (Devriendt, et al., 1997). The immune system plays a key role in the development, establishment, and progression of head and neck squamous cell carcinoma. A greater understanding of the dysregulation and evasion of the immune system in the evolution and progression provides the basis for improved therapies and outcomes for patients. Head and neck cancer cells evade the host immune system through manipulation of their own immunogenicity, production of immunosuppressive mediators, and promotion of immunomodulatory cell types (Ferris et al., 2015). Immune system dysfunction plays a role in both the development and progression of head and neck squamous cell carcinoma, highlighting the potential role for immunotherapy to improve outcomes in this disease (Ling et al., 2018; Xie, et al., 2017). Combining radiotherapy, a primary HNSCC treatment modality, with immunotherapy has been shown to induce potent antitumour immune responses in many cancers including HNSCC. In addition to its direct cytotoxic effect on the cancer cell, radiotherapy can shape the tumour microenvironment to affect the abundance and composition of tumour-infiltrating immune cells and therefore change responses to immune checkpoint inhibitor therapy (Karam et al., 2019). The immune system has a vital role in the development, establishment, and progression of head and neck squamous cell carcinoma. Immune evasion of cancer cells leads to progression of HNSCC. An understanding of this mechanism provides the basis for improved therapies and outcomes for patients. Through the tumor's influence on the microenvironment, the immune system can be exploited to promote metastasis, angiogenesis, and growth. This chapter provides an overview of the interaction between immune infiltrating cells in the tumor microenvironment, and the immunologic principles related to HNSCC. Current immunotherapeutic strategies and emerging results from ongoing clinical trials are presented (Sim et al., 2019). Head and neck squamous cell carcinomas arise in the mucosal linings of the upper aerodigestive tract and are unexpectedly heterogeneous in nature. Classical risk factors are smoking and excessive alcohol consumption, and in recent years, the role of human papillomavirus has emerged, particularly in oropharyngeal tumours (Leemans et al., 2018; Grewal et al., 2019). Literature search revealed a wide variation in dose fractionation regimens. Reported outcomes showed high efficacy and low rate of significant side effects, except in studies utilizing higher doses of radiotherapy where higher grade toxicities were seen (Iqbal et al., 2018; Zackrisson et al., 2003). The general quality of studies and the lack of information on serious side effects indicate a need for large, well-designed clinical studies with a reasonable follow-up. There is moderate evidence that patients with nasopharyngeal carcinomas of the endemic type benefit from therapy with a combination of chemotherapy and radical radiotherapy. However, the results from the reported studies are equivocal. Head and neck cancers comprise a variety of tumours depending on the sub-site, for which target volumes and the prescribed doses need to be individualized according to each patient's history and presentation. This article aims at describing the main factors involved in decision-making regarding dose and volume, as well as ongoing research (Blanchard et al., 2019). Cancer of the head and neck is a heterogeneous disease of the upper aerodigestive tract, encompassing distinct histologic types, different anatomic sites, and human papillomavirus (HPV)-positive as well as HPV-negative cancers. Advanced/recurrent HNCs have poor prognosis with low survival rates. Both are responsible for the successful escape of these tumors from the host immune system. HNCs evolve numerous mechanisms of evasion from immune destruction. These mechanisms are linked to genetic aberrations, so that HNCs with a high mutational load are also highly immunosuppressive. The tumor microenvironment of these cancers is populated by immune cells that are dysfunctional, inhibitory cytokines, and exosomes carrying suppressive ligands. Efficiency of immune therapies is expected to rapidly improve with the possibility for patients' selection based on personal immunogenomic profiles (Whiteside, 2018).

CONCLUSION

The objective of this systematic review was to identify and appraise the existing evidence of role of palliative radiotherapy for locally advanced non-metastatic head and neck cancer. A systematic search of the literature was conducted using Medline, Embase and Cochrane databases and relevant references were included.

REFERENCES

Ahn, P. H., Lukens, J. N., Boon-Keng, K. T., Kirk, M., Lin, A. The use of proton therapy in the treatment of head and neckcancers. *Cancer J.* 2014; 20(6):421-6.

Amardeep S Grewal, Joshua Jones, Alexander Lin. Palliative Radiation Therapy for Head and Neck Cancers. *Int J Radiat Oncol Biol Phys,* 2019; 105(2):254-266.

Andreassen, C. N., Eriksen, J. G., Jensen, K., Hansen, C. R., Sørensen, B. S., Lassen, P., Alsner, J., Schack, L. M. H., Overgaard, J., Grau, C.

IMRT - Biomarkers for dose escalation, dose de-escalation and personalized medicine in radiotherapy for head and neck cancer. *Oral Oncol,* 2018, 86:91-99.

Björn Zackrisson, ClaesMercke, Hans Strander, Johan Wennerberg, Eva Cavallin-Ståhl. A systematic overview of radiation therapy effects in head and neck cancer. *Acta Oncol,* 2003; 42(5-6):443-61.

Blanchard P, Baujat B, Holostenco V, Bourredjem A, Baey C, Bourhis J et al., Meta-analysis of chemotherapy in head and neck cancer (MACH-NC): a comprehensive analysis by tumour site. *Radiother Oncol* 2011, 100(1):33-40.

Bonner JA, Harari PM, Giralt J, Azarnia N, Shin DM, Cohen R B et al., Radiotherapy plus cetuximab for squamous-cell carcinoma of the head and neck. *N Engl J Med* 2006, 354(6):567-78.

Bruijnen, T., Stemkens, B., Terhaard, C. H. J., Lagendijk, J. J. W., Raaijmakers, C. P. J., Tijssen, R, H, N. Intrafraction motion quantification and planning target volume margin determination of head-and-neck tumors using cinemagnetic resonance imaging. *Radiother Oncol.* 2019, 30:82-88.

Buckmiller, L. M., Richter, G. T., Suen, J. Y. Diagnosis and management of hemangiomas and vascular malformations of the head and neck. *Oral Dis.* 2010; 16(5):405-18.

Cohen, E. E. W., Bell, R. B., Bifulco, C. B., Burtness, B., Gillison, M. L., Harrington, K. J., Le, Q. T., Lee, N. Y., Leidner, R., Lewis, R. L., Licitra, L., Mehanna, H., Mell, L. K., Raben, A., Sikora, A. G., Uppaluri, R., Whitworth, F., Zandberg, D. P., Ferris, R. L. The Society for Immunotherapy of Cancer consensus statement on immunotherapy for the treatment of squamous cell carcinoma of the head and neck (HNSCC). *J Immunother Cancer*, 2019, 7(1):184.

Czarnecka, A. M., Kukwa, W., Ścińska, A., Kukwa, A. Markery metaboliczne nowotworów głowy i szyi– aplikacje kliniczne i podłoże biochemiczne [Metabolic markers of head and neck tumors - clinical applications and biochemical background]. *Polish Otolaryngology Society.* 2009; 63 (6): 478-484.

de Bree, E., Zoras, O., Hunt, J. L., Takes, R. P., Suárez, C., Mendenhall, W. M., Hinni, M. L. Desmoid tumors of the head and neck: A therapeutic challenge. *Clinical Review*, 2014. 36(10):1517-26.

Denaro N, Russi EG, Lefebvre JL, Merlano MC. A systematic review of current and emerging approaches in the field of larynx preservation. *Radiother Oncol* 2014; 110(1):16-24.

Diane C Ling, Chris J Bakkenist, Robert L Ferris, David A Clump. Role of Immunotherapy in Head and Neck Cancer. *Semin Radiat Oncol,* 2018, 8(1):12-16.

Duffy, M. J., Crown J. A personalized approach to cancer treatment: how biomarkers can help. *Clinical Chemistry* 2008; 54 (11): 1770–1779.

Gavrielatou, N., Doumas, S., Economopoulou, P., Foukas, P. G., Psyrri, A. Biomarkers for immunotherapy response in head and neck cancer. *Cancer Treat Rev*, 2020; 84:101977.

Gronkiewicz, Z., Krzeski, A., Kukwa, W. Wybrane markery biologiczne w niektórych zmianach naczyniowych głowy i szyi. Selected biological markers in various vascular lesions of the head and neck. *Postepy Hig Med Dosw* (online), 2014; 68: 1206-1215.

Guidi, A., Codecà, C., Ferrari, D. Chemotherapy and immunotherapy for recurrent and metastatic head and neck cancer: a systematic review. *Med Oncol*, 2018, 5(3):37.

Holliday, E. B., Frank, S. T. Proton radiationtherapy for head and neck cancer: a review of the clinical experience to date. *Int J Radiat Oncol Biol Phys*, 2014, 89(2):292-302.

Kam MK, Leung SF, Zee B, Chau RM, Suen JJ, Mo F et al., Prospective randomized study of intensity-modulated radiotherapy on salivary glandfunction in early-stage nasopharyngealcarcinoma patients. *J Clin Oncol* 2007, 89(2):292-302.

Kawecki, A. Leczenie interferujące z funkcją EGFRu chorych na płaskonabłonkowegoraka narządów głowy i szyi. Anti-EGFR targeted therapy for squamos cell head and neck cancer. *Onkologia w Praktyce Klinicznej*, 2010; 6(5): 264–271.

Kemmer, J. D., Johnson, D. E., Grandis, J. R. Leveraging Genomics for Head and Neck Cancer Treatment. *J Dent Res.* 2018; 97(6): 603–613.

Magdelénat, H. Tumour markers in oncology: past, present and future. *J Immunol Methods*, 1992; 150(1-2):133-43.

Mendenhall, W. M., Dagan, R., Bryant, C. M., Fernandes, R. P. Radiation Oncology for Head and Neck Cancer: Current Standards and Future Changes. *Oral Maxillofac Surg Clin North Am*, 2019, 31(1):31-38.

Mlak, R., Krawczyk, P., Milanowski, J. Wybrane problemy kliniczne [Selected clinical problems]. *Forum Medycyny Rodzinnej* 2010; 4(2): 122–134.

Moy, J. D., Moskovitz, J. M., Ferris, R. L. Biological mechanisms of immuneescape and implications for immunotherapy in head and necks quamous cell carcinoma. *Eur J Cancer*, 2017, 76:152-166.

Nutting CM, Morden JP, Harrington KJ, Urbano TG, Bhide SA, Clark C et al., Parotid-sparing intensity modulated versus conventiona lradiotherapy in head and neck cancer (PARSPORT): aphase 3 multicentrer and omised controlled trial. *Lancet Oncol* 2011, 76:152-166.

Nutting, C. Radiotherapy in head and neck cancer management: United Kingdom National Multidisciplinary Guidelines. *The Journal of Laryngology & Otology* 2016, 130(S2):S66-S67.

René Leemans, Peter J F Snijders, Ruud H Brakenhoff. The molecular landscape of head and neck cancer. *Nat Rev Cancer*, 2018, 6(1):12.

Schoch, M., Däppen, M. B., Henke, G., Stöckli, S. Long-term sequelaeafter chemoradiation in headneck tumors. *Ther Umsch.* 2016; 73(4):213-8.

Sidharth V. Puram, James W. Rocco. Molecular Aspects of Head and Neck Cancer Therapy. *Hematol Oncol Clin North Am.* 2015; 29(6): 971–992.

Suh, Y., Amelio, I., Guerrero Urbano, T., Tavassoli, M. Clinical update on cancer: molecular oncology of head and neck cancer. *Cell Death Dis.* 2014; 5(1).

Zhu, S., Schuerch, C., Hunt, J. Review and updates of immunohistochemistry in selected salivarygland and head and neck tumors. *Arch Pathol Lab Med.* 2015 Jan; 139(1):55-66.

In: A Biochemical View of Head and Neck ... ISBN: 978-1-53619-370-1
Editors: D. Bartusik-Aebisher et al. © 2021 Nova Science Publishers, Inc.

Chapter 5

PHOTOMEDICINE OF HEAD AND NECK CANCER

Wojciech Domka, David Aebisher, Lidia Bieniasz and Dorota Bartusik-Aebisher[*]

Medical College of The University of Rzeszów

ABSTRACT

Photodynamic therapy (PDT) exploits light interactions and photosensitizers to induce cytotoxic reactive oxygen species. Photodynamic diagnosis (PDD) uses the phenomenon of photosensitizer emitting fluorescence to distinguish some tumors from normal tissue. The standard photosensitizer used for PDD is 5-aminolevulinic acid, although it is not entirely satisfactory. Many other targeted therapy strategies and medications are currently under investigation.

Keywords: photodynamic therapy, 5-ALA, cancer, photodynamic diagnosis

---

[*] Corresponding Author's Email: dbartusik-aebisher@ur.edu.pl.

The standards of radical treatment for squamous cell carcinoma of the head and neck have changed over the past decade. Compared to radiation therapy alone, this method offers significant benefits in terms of overall survival. This method is beneficial for a limited subset of patients. In this situation, it is necessary to explore new therapeutic strategies. Currently, probably the most attractive radical treatment strategy is targeted therapy combined with traditional methods such as radiotherapy or radiochemotherapy. As an information carrier, light has been developed for use in imaging, which revolutionized understanding of cancer. As an energy carrier, light has been developed for therapy, which transformed the theranostics of cancer (Li et al., 2018). Photoacoustic imaging is a noninvasive imaging modality which combines optical and ultrasound techniques. Besides conventional surgery, radiotherapy, and chemotherapy, photodynamic therapy is an alternative cancer treatment modality that induces cell death by the generation of reactive oxygen species. Photothermal reaction produces hyperthermia and coagulation of tissue; it can be an effective means in tumor tissue destruction due to the sensitivity of tumor cell to temperature elevation (Zecha et al., 2016). This could enhance patient adherence to cancer therapy, and improve quality of life and treatment outcomes (Zecha et al., 2016). Thermal ablation of tumors by Nd:YAG laser has been growing as a multidisciplinary subspecialty defined as laser-induced thermal therapy, and has been increasingly accepted as a minimally invasive method for palliation of advanced or recurrent cancer. Previous studies have shown that adjuvant chemotherapy can potentiate laser thermal ablation of tumors leading to improved palliation in advanced cancer patients (Palumbo et al., 2017; Khachemoune et al., 2005). Photodynamic therapy was discovered more than 100 years ago, and has since become a well-studied therapy for cancer and various non-malignant diseases including infections. Photodynamic Therapy (PDT) uses photosensitizers that are activated by absorption of visible light to initially form the excited singlet state, followed by transition to the long-lived excited triplet state (Abrahamse et al., 2016). Photodynamic therapy is a promising modality for the treatment of cancer. The reactive oxygen species produced during PDT are responsible for the oxidation of biomolecules, which in turn cause cell death and the necrosis of malignant tissue compounds with photosensitizing activity have been introduced commercially (Mansoori et al., 2019). The most common significant adverse event after photodynamic therapy with porfimer sodium is esophageal stricture formation. This study assessed whether pretreatment variables, including prior endoscopic therapy for Barrett's esophagus, are associated with post-PDT stricturing. An increased risk of stricture development was seen after multiple courses of PDT (Yachimski et al., 2008). Head and neck squamous cell carcinomas are an aggressive, genetically complex and difficult to treat group of cancers (Alsahafi et al., 2019). PDT proves its value in treatment of patients with field cancerization and patients with superficial recurrence after previous surgery and/or radiation, in whom surgical salvage would entail important morbidity. PDT is also promising as an adjuvant treatment after surgery in the presence of macroscopic or microscopic involved margins, in patients where reresection or reirradiation would imply an unacceptable risk. Photodynamic therapy, a treatment of choice for cancer, induces a photochemical reaction, thereby eradicating tumor cells. However, its adverse events and complicated procedure and the development of alternative endoscopic procedures such as endoscopic submucosal dissection, radiofrequency ablation and cryotherapy, have largely limited the practice of PDT in esophageal cancer worldwide (Wu et al., 2019). There was previously reported that photodynamic therapy induces cell death in head and neck cancer through both autophagy and apoptosis. However, the mechanism is still unclear (Kim et al., 2016). NF-κB expression was detected by an electrophoretic mobility shift assay, hypoxia-inducible factor α (HIF-1α) and vascular endothelial growth factor (VEGF) by real-time PCR, NF-κB, HIF-1α, and VEGF protein by western blot, and Ki-67, HIF-1α, VEGF, and NF-κB protein by immunohistochemistry. PDT increased NF-κB activity and the gene expression of HIF-1α and VEGF *in vitro* and *in vivo* (Driehuis et al., 2019). Patients diagnosed with head and neck squamous cell carcinoma) are currently treated with surgery and/or radio- and chemotherapy. In photodynamic therapy, a light-activated photosensitizer produces reactive oxygen species that ultimately lead to cell death. Targeted PDT, using a photosensitizer conjugated to tumor-targeting molecules, has been explored as a more selective cancer therapy (van Doeveren et al., 2018). In case of close or positive resection margins after oncological resection in head and neck surgery, additional treatment is necessary. When conventional options are exhausted, photodynamic therapy can play a role in achieving clear margins. The purpose of the current study was to evaluate the clinical benefit of PDT as adjuvant therapy next to surgery with positive resection margins. Overall, results show that these EGFR targeted nanobody-PS conjugates are selective and able to induce tumor cell death *in vivo*. Additional studies are now needed to assess the full potential of this approach to improving PDT (van Driel et al., 2016). Photodynamic therapy (PDT) utilizes a sensitizer agent and light to produce selective cell death. Dermatologists are familiar with PDT for the treatment of actinic keratoses and early nonmelanoma skin cancers, and recent studies have elucidated that PDT has resulted in improved morbidity and secondary outcomes for the treatment of various cancerous and precancerous solid tumors. Light source and dosimetry may be modified to selectively target tissue, and novel techniques such as fractionation, metronomic pulsation, continuous light delivery, and chemophototherapy are under investigation for further optimization of therapy. This article aims to review the expanding indications for PDT and demonstrate the potential of this modality to decrease morbidity and increase quality of life for patients. Data on efficacy, survival, and side effects vary across tumor types but support PDT for the treatment of numerous solid tumors. With new advances in PDT, indications for this therapeutic modality may expand (Yanovsky et al., 2019; Shafirstein et al., 2018). The significance of percutaneous dilatational tracheostomy in combination with tumour surgery of the head neck area has not yet been fully considered (Knipping et al., 2016; Shi, et al., 2018). Esophageal cancer is a common gastrointestinal cancer viability was measured by MTT assay and cell apoptosis was determined by Annexin V-PE/7-AAD and western blot. A set of five human cancer cell lines from head and neck and other PDT-relevant tissues was used to investigate oxidative stress and underlying cell death mechanisms of mTHPC-mediated PDT *in vitro*. In general, the overall phototoxic effects and the concentrations as well as the time to establish these effects varies between cell lines, suggesting that the cancer cells are not all dying by one defined mechanism, but rather succumb to an individual interplay of different cell death mechanisms. Besides the evaluation of the underlying cell death mechanisms, authors focused on the comparison of results in a set of five identically treated cell lines in this study. Although cells were treated under equitoxic conditions and PDT acts via a rather unspecific ROS formation, very heterogeneous results were obtained with different cell lines. This study shows that general conclusions after PDT *in vitro* require testing on several cell lines to be reliable, which has too often been ignored in the past (Zhu et al., 2019). The noninvasive nature of photodynamic therapy enables the preservation of organ function in cancer patients. However, PDT is impeded by hypoxia in the tumor microenvironment caused by high intracellular oxygen consumption and distorted tumor blood vessels. Therefore, increasing oxygen generation in the TME would be a promising methodology for enhancing PDT. Herein, the authors proposed a concept of ferroptosis promoted PDT based on the biochemical characteristics of cellular ferroptosis, which improved the PDT efficacy significantly by producing reactive oxygen species (ROS) and supplying O2 sustainably through the Fenton reaction (Kweon et al., 2016). To evaluate the functional characteristics of swallowing and to analyze the parameters of dysphagia in head and neck cancer patients after concurrent chemoradiotherapy. The medical records of 32 patients with head and neck cancer who were referred for a videofluoroscopic swallowing study from January 2012 to May 2015 were retrospectively reviewed. Therefore, swallowing therapy targeting the pharyngeal phase is recommended after CCRT (Liu et al., 2019). Photodynamic therapy using δ-aminolevulinic acid photosensitization has shown promise in clinical studies for the treatment of early-stage oral malignancies with fewer potential side effects than traditional therapies. Light delivery to oral lesions can also carried out with limited medical infrastructure suggesting the potential for implementation of PDT in global health settings. The authors sought to develop a cost-effective, battery-powered, fiber-coupled PDT system suitable for intraoral light delivery enabled by smartphone interface and embedded electronics for ease of operation. Device performance was assessed in measurements of optical power output, spectral stability, and preclinical assessment of PDT response in ALA-photosensitized squamous carcinoma cell cultures and murine subcutaneous tumor xenografts. The device has a compact configuration, user friendly operation and flexible light delivery for the oral cavity. *In vivo* PDT response (reduction in tumor volume) is comparable with a commercial 635 nm laser. The authors developed a low-cost, LED-based, fiber-coupled PDT light delivery source that has stable output on battery power and suitable form factor for deployment in rural and/or resource-limited settings. Photodynamic therapy is a minimally invasive treatment for malignant tumors. The aim of this study was to determine the efficacy of PDT in patients with head and neck squamous cell carcinoma (Hosokawa et al., 2018). PDT is an effective therapy to treat HNSCC, and leads to an improved quality of life in patients with residual or recurrent disease (Civantos et al., 2018). Photodynamic therapy involves the use of a phototoxic drug which is activated by low powered laser light to destroy neoplastic cells. Multiple photosensitizers have been studied and tumors have been treated in a variety of head and neck sites over the last 30 years. PDT can effectively treat head and neck tumors, particularly those of the superficial spreading type, and the classic application of this technology has been in the patient with a wide field of dysplastic change and superficial carcinomatosis. This study aimed to further investigate the possible molecular mechanism underlying the effect of ALA-PDT (Fang et al., 2018). Photodynamic therapy is generally safer and less invasive than conventional strategies for head and neck cancer treatment. However, currently available photosensitizers have low selectivity for tumor cells, and the burden and side effects are so great that research is needed to develop safe photosensitizers. In this study, it was confirmed that the Buddleja officinalis extract, used in the treatment of inflammation and vascular diseases, shows fluorescence when activated by LED light, and, based on this, The authors aimed to develop a new photosensitive agent suitable for PDT (Cho et al., 2018). One such alternative anticancer approach is known as photodynamic therapy (PDT), where a non-toxic photosensitizer produces oxidative stress via the formation of reactive oxygen species after local illumination of the affected tissue. A very promising PS is 5,10,15,20-tetra(m-hydroxyphenyl)chlorin (mTHPC, Temoporfin), which is approved for the treatment of head and neck cancer in Europe. Cytotoxicity was determined by the MTT assay and synergistic effects on cytotoxicity were evaluated by calculation of Combination Indices. Synergy was identified in some of the combinations, for example, with 1-OHP in three of the tested cell lines but antagonism was also observed for a number of combinations in certain cell lines. In cases of synergy, elevated ROS levels were observed after combination but apoptosis induction was not necessarily increased compared to a treatment with a single compound (Lange et al., 2018). Photodynamic therapy is a clinically approved cancer therapy, based on a photochemical reaction between a light activatable molecule or photosensitizer, light, and molecular oxygen. When these three harmless components are present together, reactive oxygen species are formed. Since its regulatory approval, over 30 years ago, PDT has been the subject of numerous studies and has proven to be an effective form of cancer therapy. This review provides an overview of the clinical trials conducted over the last 10 years, illustrating how PDT is applied in the clinic today. Furthermore, examples from ongoing clinical trials and the most recent preclinical studies are presented, to show the directions, in which PDT is headed, in the near and distant future. Despite the clinical success reported, PDT is still currently underutilized in the clinic. The authors also discuss the factors that hamper the exploration of this effective therapy and what should be changed to render it a more effective and more widely available option for patients (van Straten et al., 2017). Photodynamic therapy investigations have seen stable increases and the development of new photosensitizers is a heated topic. Sinoporphyrin sodium is a new photosensitizer isolated from Photofrin (Shi et al., 2017). Photodynamic therapy is a palliative treatment option for head and neck squamous cell carcinoma patients which induces local inflammation and alters tumor cell morphology. The PDT-mediated conversion from the mesenchymal to epithelial tumor phenotype was mediated by exosomes, which also served as non-invasive biomarkers of this transition (Theodoraki et al., 2018; Li et al., 2019). PDT appears to be a useful therapeutic strategy in the management of oral leukoplakia as a non-surgical treatment (Marchal et al., 2015). Through the combination of a photosensitizing agent with light and oxygen, PDT produces highly cytotoxic reactive oxygen species leading to selective tumor eradication. PDT is an attractive treatment for focal therapy of localized tumors, especially in the case of unresectable tumors. In HNSCC, over 1500 patients have been treated by PDT, and the majority of them responded quite favorably to this treatment. Photodynamic therapy represents a palliative treatment resulting in induction of inflammatory reactions with importance for the development of an antitumor immunity. Cancer/testis antigens have been associated with poor prognosis in different types of cancer, including head and neck squamous cell carcinoma. The authors investigated vandetanib, which selectively blocks EGFR and vascular endothelial growth factor receptor-2, to enhance the efficacy of PDT. The authors assessed the *in vitro* therapeutic efficacy of: 1) vandetanib; 2) PDT with the photosensitizer Chlorin e6 combined PDT + vadetanib treatment in CAL-27 oral squamous cell carcinoma cell line by cell viability, γH2AX foci immunostaining, cell cycle arrest and western blot (Chu et al., 2019). PDT resulted in significant tumour growth delay *in vivo* that is linked to reduction of PDT-induced EGFR phosphorylation and cellular proliferation, along with loss of tumour vasculature (Farrakhova et al., 2019). This article presents the results of intraoperative fluorescent diagnostics via the endoscopic system for assessing the quality of photodynamic therapy of head and neck cancer. The diagnosis and PDT procedures were performed on the five patients with malignant neoplasms of the vocal cords, lateral surface of the tongue, and trachea and cancer of the left parotid salivary gland. Fluorescent diagnostics was conducted before PDT and after PDT procedures. Control of PDT efficiency was carried out by evaluating the photobleaching of the drug. The method of intraoperative fluorescent imaging allows determining the exact location of the tumor and its boundaries. The assessment of photosensitizer photobleaching in real time regime allows making quick decisions during

PDT procedure, which helps improving the quality of patients' treatment. Therefore, this diagnostic approach will improve the effectiveness of cancer treatment. To assess the impact of photodynamic therapy parameters in the management of oral potentially malignant disorders (Jin et al., 2019).

5-Aminolevulinic acid is a prodrug used in photodynamic therapy of tumors, including cancer of the oral mucosa. 5-ALA poorly penetrates oral tissues due to its high hydrophilicity, which impairs its local effects in PDT. The *in vitro* release profiles of the selected formulation and its respective control were determined using artificial membranes (Quintanilha et al., 2017). Photodynamic therapy represents a palliative treatment option for a selected group of patients with head and neck squamous cell carcinoma. Serum concentrations of T cell related cytokine panel, including HMGB1, IL-6, IL-10 and perforin were measured by bead array and ELISA (Quintanilha et al., 2017). In heavily pretreated HNSCC patients, the number and frequency of Treg and NK-cells were increased as compared to NC. PDT induced a further increase of the frequency of Treg and NK-cells in the peripheral blood. Additionally, the serum concentrations of HMGB1, IL-6 and IL-10 showed a significant elevation after treatment with simultaneously decreased perforin levels (Quintanilha et al., 2017). Although PDT is a local treatment regimen, a systemic inflammatory response with altered peripheral immune cell populations and cytokine concentrations is visible. The increased Treg and NK cell numbers after PDT support the hypothesis that PDT may successfully be combined with NK cell or T cell activating immune checkpoint modulators in HNSCC patients to improve HNSCC specific immunity (Gan et al., 2020). To investigate whether the Warburg effect is a key modulator on the resistance mechanism of photodynamic therapy. Glycolysis was examined by the test of lactate product and glucose uptake at different post-PDT time points. Cell viability was detected by the CCK-8 assay and cell proliferation was detected by colony formation assay. The combined treatment of 2-DG and PDT significantly inhibited tumor growth *in vitro* at 24 h. (Quintanilha et al., 2017). Photodynamic therapy is a therapeutic alternative for malignant tumors that uses a photosensitizer. These data demonstrate that HYP could be an effective photosensitizer for human ATC therapy (Kim et al., 2018). Photodynamic therapy and photothermal therapy using nanoparticles have gained significant attention for its therapeutic effect for cancer treatment. In the present study, the authors fabricated polypyrrole nanoparticles by employing bovine serum albumin-phycocyanin complex and the formulated particles were stable in various physiological solutions like water, phosphate buffered saline and culture media (Bharathiraja et al., 2018). Efficacy of ionizing radiation (I/R) was compared with phototoxic effects of photodynamic therapy *in vitro* using two cell lines derived from patients with head and neck squamous cell carcinoma (Kessel et al., 2020). Multiple clinical studies have shown that interstitial photodynamic therapy is a promising modality in the treatment of locally-advanced cancerous tumors. However, the utilization of I-PDT has been limited to several centers. The objective of this focused review is to highlight the different approaches employed to administer I-PDT with photosensitizers that are either approved or in clinical studies for the treatment of prostate cancer, pancreatic cancer, head and neck cancer, and brain cancer (Shafirstein et al., 2017). The aim of the present study was to systematically review the efficacy of photodynamic therapy in the management of oral potentially-malignant disorders (PMDS) and head and neck squamous cell carcinoma. Review articles, experimental studies, case reports, commentaries, letters to the editor, unpublished articles, and articles published in languages other than English were excluded (Gondivkar et al., 2018). Photosensitizers used were aminolevulinic acid, meta-tetrahydroxyphenylchlorin, Foscan, hematoporphyrin derivatives, Photofrin, Photosan, and chlorine-e6. Laser wavelength, power density, irradiation duration were 585-652 nm, 50-500 mW/cm2, and 1-143 minutes, respectively. High expression of secreted protein acidic and rich in cysteine in oral squamous cell cancer and CAFs was also confirmed in study (Wang et al., 2019). Photodynamic therapy is a salvage treatment for local failure following chemoradiotherapy for esophageal cancer. L-PDT represented better short-term outcomes than P-PDT as a salvage treatment for local failure following CRT or RT for esophageal cancer (Minamide et al., 2020). Sulforaphene a natural isothiocyanate from cruciferous vegetables has shown a potential anticancer effect against cervical and lung cancer. Palliative treatments like photodynamic therapy are being implemented for a long time however, the results are still not promising in case of aggressive cancers like anaplastic thyroid cancer. PDT against anaplastic thyroid cancer (Chatterjee et al., 2018). The low survival rate of head and neck cancer (HNC) patients is attributable to late disease diagnosis and high recurrence rate. Current HNC staging has inadequate accuracy and low sensitivity for effective diagnosis and treatment management. The multimodal porphyrin lipoprotein-mimicking nanoparticle, intrinsically capable of positron emission tomography (PET), fluorescence imaging, and photodynamic therapy (PDT), shows great potential to enhance the accuracy of HNC staging and potentially HNC management (Muhanna, et al., 2016). Photodynamic therapy has been considered to be a possible candidate approach for the treatment of multidrug-resistant cancer. Histopathology was also used to confirm this antitumor effect (Kim et al., 2016). Greatly prolonged survival of rabbits is observed after such intraluminal PDT treatment (Xiao et al., 2019). Drug resistance remains a formidable challenge to cancer therapy. The main reason for the failure is lack of cancer specificity of small-molecule Pgp inhibitors, thus causing severe toxicity in normal tissues. *In vitro* studies showed that the antibody-photosensitizer conjugates specifically bind to Pgp-expressing drug resistant cancer cells, and caused dramatic cytotoxicity upon irradiation with a near infrared light (Mao et al., 2018). As irreplaceable energy sources of minimally invasive treatment, light and sound have, separately, laid solid foundations in their clinic applications. Constrained by the relatively shallow penetration depth of light, photodynamic therapy typically involves involves superficial targets such as shallow seated skin conditions, head and neck cancers, eye disorders, early-stage cancer of esophagus, etc. For ultrasound-driven sonodynamic therapy, however, to various organs is facilitated by the superior... transmission and focusing ability of ultrasound in biological tissues, enabling multiple therapeutic applications including treating glioma, breast cancer, hematologic tumor and opening blood-brain-barrier. The therapeutic dynamics and current designs of pharmacological sensitizers involved in these therapies are presented (Yang et al., 2019). With recent developments in photosensitizers and light delivery systems, topical 5-aminolevulinic acid-mediated photodynamic therapy has become the fourth alternative therapeutic approach in the management of oral leucoplakia due to its minimally invasive nature, efficacy, and low risk of systemic side effects and disfigurement (Chen et al., 2019). The incidence of differentiated thyroid cancer has increased significantly during the last several decades. Photodynamic therapy has the potential to reduce treatment-related side effects by decreasing invasiveness and limiting toxicity. This resulted in significant and specific apoptosis in tumor tissue, but not surrounding normal tissues including trachea and recurrent laryngeal nerve. A long-term survival study further demonstrated that PLP-PDT enabled complete ablation of tumor tissue while sparing both the normal thyroid tissue and RLN from damage, thus providing a safe, minimally invasive, and effective alternative to thyroidectomy for thyroid cancer therapies (Muhanna et al., 2020). Image-based treatment planning can be used to compute the delivered light dose during interstitial photodynamic therapy of locally advanced head and neck squamous cell carcinoma. The objectives of this work were to evaluate the use of surface fiducial markers and flexible adhesive grids in guiding interstitial placement of laser fibers, and to quantify the impact of discrepancies in fiber location on the expected light dose volume histograms. Clinical flexible grids and fiducial markers were used to guide the insertion of optically transparent catheters, which are used to place cylindrical diffuser fibers within the phantoms. There was a statistically significant difference between all seven phantoms in terms of the mean displacement. There was also statistically significant correlation between DVHs and depth of insertion, but not with the lateral displacement. The maximum difference between actual and planned DVH was related to the number of fibers and the treatment time (Oakley et al., 2017). Photodynamic therapy is suggested to have an impact on the treatment of early stage head and neck cancers. The authors investigated the effect of PDT with methylene blue and a diode laser (660 nm) as the laser source on HNSCC cell lines as an *in vitro* model of surface oral squamous cell carcinoma. Cell-cultures were exposed to 160 µM MB for 4 min and to laser light for 8 min. Viability was proven via cell viability assay and clonogenic survival via clone counting assay (Kofler et al., 2018). Photodynamic therapy is believed to promote hypoxic conditions to tumor cells leading to overexpression of angiogenic markers such as vascular endothelial growth factor. Topical methyl aminolevulinate photodynamic therapy (MAL-PDT) with 3 h incubation is recommended as a field directed treatment. Skin pretreatment with ablative CO2 fractional laser prior to MAL-PDT enhances drug penetration and could minimize incubation time. To evaluate and compare the safety and the preventive effect in the development of new non-melanocytic skin cancers of AFXL-assisted MAL-PDT with 1-h incubation with that of conventional MAL-PDT in patients with clinical and histological signs of field cancerization. Forty-two patients with two mirror cancerized areas of face or scalp were randomized to field treatment with 1-h incubation AFXL-assisted PDT or conventional PDT. All patients underwent two treatment sessions 1 week apart. Irradiation was performed using a red light-emitting diode lamp at 37 J/cm2. All patients completed the study. There was no statistically significant difference with respect to the total number of new actinic keratoses at any point of follow-up as well as to the mean time of occurrence of new lesions between treatment fields. Both treatment regimens were safe and well tolerated (Vrani et al., 2019). Ablative CO2 fractional laser pretreatment may be considered as an option for reducing photosensitizer occlusion time while providing the same preventative efficacy as CPDT in patients with field-cancerized skin (Vrani et al., 2019). Laryngeal diseases are closely related to the swallowing and speech function of the patients. Protecting and restoring laryngeal function, while curing lesions, is vital to patients' quality of life. Photodynamic therapy (PDT) is a minimally invasive method which is widely used in the treatment of tumor, precancerous lesions, and inflammatory diseases. In recent years, it has been shown to have a protective effect on normal structures. This article reviews the clinical outcomes of laryngeal diseases treated with PDT since 1990 in order to evaluate its efficacy and significance. The prolonged adverse effects of the first-generation photosensitizers have limited the application of PDT. With the improvement of photosensitizers and treatment strategies, PDT promises to be a safe, effective, and minimally invasive treatment method for laryngeal diseases (Zhang et al., 2018). Photodynamic therapy is a nonsurgical, minimally invasive treatment that uses a light source to activate light-sensitive drugs or photosensitizers in the treatment of cancer and other diseases. PDT has been successfully employed to treat early carcinomas of the oral cavity and larynx preserving normal tissue and vital functions of speech and swallowing (Abramson et al., 1994). Twenty-four hours prior to photoactivation, patients received 2.5 mg/kg of dihematoporphyrin ether intravenously. Photodynamic therapy was given using an argon pump dye laser system (Abramson et al., 1994; Kavuru et al., 1990). Photodynamic therapy (PDT), might be as effective for and better tolerated by the patients concerned.

PDT is a highly effective method to treat head and neck (pre)malignancies. Nevertheless, further clinical studies are needed to better define its true value in head and neck oncology (Volgger et al., 2016; Rosin et al., 2019).

Photodynamic therapy (PDT), an O2-dependent treatment for inhibition of cancer proliferation, suffers from the low therapeutic effect in clinical application due to the hypoxic microenvironment in tumor cells (Shen et al., 2017; Ahn et al., 2018). Measurement of the physiologic properties of target lesions may allow for identification of patients with the highest probability of benefiting from PDT. This provides opportunity for optimizing light delivery based on lesion characteristics and/or informing ongoing clinical decision-making in patients who would most benefit from PDT. Despite excellent healing of the oral mucosa in PDT, a lack of robust enabling technology for intraoral light delivery has limited its broader implementation (Mallidi et al., 2019). Oral cancer is a serious public health issue. Apart from its high rate of prevalence, incidence and mortality, it can often result in more complex and expensive treatment when diagnosed late. Potentially malignant disorders can precede oral cancer, and are usually treated by surgical excision. However, in many cases patients are elderly and multiple interventions may be required. Due to the lack of standardization regarding photosensitizers, types of irradiation, and methods of application, the objective of this study was to analyze existing PDT protocols in an attempt to identify the one that demonstrates greater efficiency, reliability and feasibility in the treatment of oral PMDs for both researchers and clinicians (Figueira, et al., 2017). Photodynamic therapy is used to treat early proximal bronchial cancer during a flexible bronchoscopy. The technique relies on the excitation of a photosensitizer by an appropriate wavelength, which is delivered into the bronchus in close contact with the tumor. To assess methylene blue as a PDT agent for the treatment of respiratory tract cancer in animal models (Obstoy et al., 2016). Photodynamic therapy for Barrett's esophagus and dysplasia are achieving dramatic initial results. Although the long-term efficacy of these nonspecific ablative therapies is awaiting longitudinal studies, reports of recurrences are increasing (Xian et al., 2019). Advanced head and neck squamous cell carcinoma, after locoregional treatment and multiple lines of systemic therapies, represents a great challenge to overcome acquired resistance. The present clinical case illustrates a successful treatment option and is the first to describe the use of photodynamic therapy with Redaporfin, followed by immune checkpoint inhibition with an anti-PD1 antibody. This patient presented an extensive tumor in the mouth pavement progressing after surgery, radiotherapy, and multiple lines of systemic treatment. PDT with Redaporfin achieved the destruction of all visible tumor, and the sequential use of an immune checkpoint inhibitor allowed a sustained complete response (Santos et al., 2018). Photodynamic therapy has been indicated for oral squamous cell carcinoma at early stages. Further studies are necessary to confirm whether this PDT-resistance phenotype can be clinically present, mainly in OSCC showing clinical recurrences after exposure to different PDT protocols (Rosin et al., 2018). Photodynamic therapy is a minimally invasive treatment option for early esophageal cancer. Among these genes, both tumor necrosis factor (TNF) and EFNA1 genes were significantly upregulated in resistant cell lines (Yang et al., 2015). The authors previously reported glucose-conjugated chlorin as a more effective photosensitizer than another widely used photosensitizer, talaporfin sodium (TS); however, G-chlorin is hydrophobic. Authors synthesized oligosaccharide-conjugated chlorin (O-chlorin) with improved water-solubility (Nishie et al., 2016). In this study, authors applied photoacoustic imaging to visualize the depth distribution of ICG-lactosome in a mouse subcutaneous tumor model. These results show the usefulness of PA imaging for monitoring not only photosensitizer accumulation and bleaching but also vascular responses in PDT with ICG-lactosome. This method can be applied to the diagnosis of many types of PDT processes (Tsunoi et al., 2019). Individuals with medical history of non-melanoma skin cancers (NMSCs) usually develop multiple and/or recurrent malignant lesions around the site of the primary neoplasm. The latter represents the clinical expression of the 'field cancerization' theory; supporting the presence of multiple malignant clones of dysplastic keratinocytes over the entire epithelium that potentially can progress into clinical lesions. Cellular uptake, cytotoxicity, intracellular location, biodistribution and antitumor effects were studied using human esophageal cancer cells (Eca-109) and human cervical cancer cells (Hela) *in vitro* and an esophageal cancer model in BALB/c nude mice. Cellular uptake and biodistribution of TMC were measured by fluorescence spectrophotometer. (Zhang et al., 2016; Liang et al., 2019; Korbelik et al., 2019). Targeted photodynamic therapy in head/neck cancer patients with a conjugate of the anti-epidermal growth factor receptor (EGFR) antibody, Cetuximab and a phthalocyanine photosensitizer IR700DX is under way, but the exact mechanisms of action are still not fully understood (Peng et al., 2020). Despite the advantages of using photodynamic therapy for the treatment of head and neck tumors, it can only be used to treat early stage flat lesions due to the limited tissue penetration ability of the visible light (Mao et al., 2016). Management of early superficial lesions in the head and neck remains complex (Ahn et al., 2016). PDT was delivered to 30/35 subjects, with 29 evaluable. There was one death possibly due to the treatment. The regimen was otherwise tolerable, with a 52% rate of grade 3 mucositis which healed within several weeks. Photodynamic therapy and esophageal stent implantation in improving dysphagia caused by malignant obstruction of middle and advanced esophageal cancer (Ding et al., 2020). The authors have shown that stresses, including photodynamic therapy, can disrupt the de novo sphingolipid biosynthesis pathway, leading to changes in the levels of sphingolipids, and subsequently, modulation of cell death (Boppana et al., 2016). This study investigated whether diffuse optical spectroscopy (DOS) measurements could assess clinical response to photodynamic therapy in patients with head and neck squamous cell carcinoma (HNSCC) (Rohrbach et al., 2016). Photodynamic therapy has shown promise in the treatment of early head and neck squamous cell carcinoma. In photodynamic therapy a light sensitive drug and visible light cause cancer cell death by the creation of singlet oxygen and free radicals, inciting an immune response, and vascular collapse. In this paper, authors review several studies that demonstrate the effectiveness of PDT in the treatment of early stage SCC of the head and neck, with some showing a similar response rate to surgery. Two cases are presented to illustrate the effectiveness of PDT. Then, new advances are discussed including the discovery of STAT3 crosslinking as a potential biomarker for PDT response and interstitial PDT for locally advanced cancers (Mimikos et al., 2016; Shafirstein et al., 2016).

To evaluate the effectiveness of photodynamic therapy in the management of choroidal metastasis (Ghodasra et al., 2016). Photodynamic therapy may be an effective therapeutic option for the management of choroidal metastasis in selected cases. To assess the effect of photodynamic therapy with talaporfin sodium, a second-generation photosensitizer, on oral squamous cell carcinoma (Pramual et al., 2017; Qiao et al., 2016). Photodynamic therapy is a highly localized and minimally invasive cancer treatment modality with many important advantages, but the lack of ideal photosensitizers greatly restricts its clinical utility. To develop new PSs with highly efficient singlet oxygen production and high tumor-localizing ability to reduce damage to healthy adjacent tissues, authors conjugated folic acid with pyropheophorbide a potent PS with a very high singlet oxygen quantum yield and a high extinction coefficient (Wang et al., 2017). Photodynamic therapy is a procedure based on the interaction between a photosensitizer, a light source with a specific wavelength and oxygen (Grandi et al., 2018; Liu et al., 2018). Acid ceramidase has been identified as a promising target for cancer therapy (Korbelik et al., 2016). Photodynamic therapy is a relatively new method of treating various kinds of pathologies. Comparisons with the clinical features, rate of recurrence and overall outcome were made (Jerjes et al., 2017). The technique is simple, can commonly be carried out in outpatient clinics, and is highly acceptable to patients. Interestingly, sequential combination therapy enhances the anticancer efficacy of drugs like cisplatin via synergistic effects (Xue et al., 2019). Fluorescence emission, cell viability, and intracellular distribution of candidates were analyzed to screen potential photosensitizers from traditional plant extracts (Shi et al., 2019). Photodynamic therapy of head and neck squamous cell carcinomas. Thus, these results make these micelles a promising nanomedicine formulation for selective therapy (Liu et al., 2020). In retrospective study, a total of 62 patients with actinic keratosis were treated with surface illumination PDT. Comparisons with the clinical features, rate of recurrence as well as malignant transformation and overall outcome were made (Jerjes et al., 2017; Kessels et al., 2016). The development of agents for noninvasive photothermal/photodynamic therapies against cancer remains challenging because most PTT agents cause side effects on normal tissues due to their high cytotoxicity and slow metabolism rate. The combination of these hypotoxic and metabolic hybrid nanoparticles with radiation therapy has potential for the future treatment of OSCC (Ren et al., 2017). The photophysical and cellular properties of TDPP were investigated (Li et al., 2015).

Conclusion

Photodynamic therapy is a minimally invasive intervention used in the management of tissue disorders. Tumor drug resistance limits the response to chemotherapy. Selective accumulation of photosensitizers into cancerous cells is one of the most important factors affecting photodynamic therapy efficacy.

REFERENCES

Abrahamse, H; Hamblin, MR. New photosensitizers for photodynamictherapy. *Biochem J*, 2016, 473(4), 347–364.

Abramson, AL; Shikowitz, MJ; Mullooly, VM; Steinberg, BM; Hyman, RB. Variable light-dose effect on photodynamic therapy for laryngeal papillomas. *Arch Otolaryngol Head Neck Surg*, 1994, 120(8), 852-5.

Ahn, MY; Yoon, HE; Moon, SY; Kim, YC; Yoon, JH. Intratumoral Photodynamic Therapy With Newly Synthesized Pheophorbide a in Murine Oral Cancer. *Oncol Res*, 2017, 25(2), 295-304.

Ahn, PH; Finlay, JC; Gallagher-Colombo, SM; Quon, H; O'Malley, Jr. BW; Weinstein, GS; Chalian, A; Malloy, K; Sollecito, T; Greenberg, M; Simone, 2nd. CB; McNulty, S; Lin, A; Zhu, T. C; Livolsi, V; Feldman, M; Mick, R; Cengel, KA; Busch, TM. Lesion oxygenation associates with clinical outcomes in premalignant and early stage head and neck tumors treated on a phase 1 trial of photodynamic therapy. *Photodiagnosis Photodyn Ther*, 2018, 21, 28-35.

Ahn, PH; Quon, H; W O'Malley, B; Weinstein, G; Chalian, A; Malloy, K; Atkins, J. H; Sollecito, T; Greenberg, M; McNulty, S; Lin, A; Zhu, TC; Finlay, JC; Cengel, K. Virginia Livolsi 8, Michael Feldman 8, Rosemarie Mick 9, Theresa M Busch. Toxicities and early outcomes in a phase 1 trial of photodynamic therapy for premalignant and early stage head and neck tumors. *Oral Oncol*, 2016, 55, 37-42.

Akbarzadeh, F; Khoshgard, K; Arkan, E; Hosseinzadeh, L; Azandaryani, AH. Evaluating the photodynamic therapy efficacy using 5-aminolevulinic acid and folic acid-conjugated bismuth oxide nanoparticles on human nasopharyngeal carcinoma cell line. *Artif Cells Nanomed Biotechnol*, 2018, 46(sup3), S514-S523.

Alsahafi, E; Begg, K; Amelio, I; Raulf, N; Lucarelli, P; Sauter, T; Tavassoli, M. Clinical update on head and neck cancer: molecular biology and ongoing challenges Alsahafi et al. *Cell Death and Disease*, 2019, 10, 540.

Bharathiraja, S; Panchanathan Manivasagan, Madhappan Santha Moorthy, Nhat Quang Bui, Bian Jang, Thi Tuong Vy Phan, Won-Kyo Jung,

Young-Mok Kim, Kang Dae Lee, Junghwan Oh. Photo-based PDT/PTT dual model killing and imaging of cancer cells using phycocyanin-polypyrrole nanoparticles. *Eur J Pharm Biopharm*, 2018, 123, 20-30.

Biel, M4A. Photodynamic therapy treatment of early oral and laryngeal cancers. *Photochem Photobiol*, 2007, 8 3(5), 1063-8.

Boppana, NB; DeLor, JS; Van Buren, E; Bielawska, A; Bielawski, J; Pierce, JS; Korbelik, M; Separovic, D. Enhanced apoptotic cancer cell killing after Foscan photodynamic therapy combined with fenretinide via de novo sphingolipid biosynthesis pathway. *J Photochem Photobiol B*, 2016, 159, 191-5.

Chatterjee, S; Rhee, Y; Chung, PS; Ge, RF; Ahn, JC. Sulforaphene Enhances The Efficacy of Photodynamic Therapy In Anaplastic Thyroid Cancer Through Ras/RAF/MEK/ERK Pathway Suppression. *J Photochem Photobiol B*, 2018, 179, 46-53.

Chen, Q; Dan, H; Tang, F; Wang, J; Li, X; Cheng, J; Zhao, H; Zeng, X. Photodynamic therapy guidelines for the management of oral leucoplakia. *Int J Oral Sci*, 2019, 11(2), 14.

Cho, H; Zheng, H; Sun, Q; Shi, S; He, Y; Ahn, K; Kim, B; Kim, HE; Kim, O. Development of Novel Photosensitizer Using the Buddleja officinalis Extract for Head and Neck Cancer. *Evid Based Complement Alternat Med*, 2018, 2018, 6917590.

Chu, PL; Shihabuddeen, WA; Low, KP; Poon, DJJ; Ramaswamy, B; Liang, ZG; Nei, WL; Chua, KLM; Thong, PSP; Soo, KC; Yeo, ELL; Chua, MLK. Vandetanib sensitizes head and neck squamous cell carcinoma to photodynamic therapy through modulation of EGFR-dependent DNA repair and the tumour microenvironment. *Photodiagnosis Photodyn Ther*, 2019, 27, 367-374.

Civantos, FJ; Karakullukcu, B; Biel, M; Silver, CE; Rinaldo, A; Saba, NF; Takes, RP; Poorten, VV; Ferlito, A. A Review of Photodynamic Therapy for Neoplasms of the Head and Neck. *Adv Ther*, 2018, 35(3), 324-340.

Ding, Y; Li, W; Li, B; Zhang, W; Peng, LJ; Bai, NF; Hu, XK. [Comparison between photodynamic therapy and interventional esophageal stent implantation in dysphagia caused by advanced esophageal cancer]. *Zhonghua Yi Xue Za Zhi*, 2020, 100(5), 378-381.

Driehuis, E; Spelier, S; Hernández, IB; de Bree, R; Willems, SM; Clevers, H; Oliveira, S. Patient-Derived Head and Neck Cancer Organoids Recapitulate EGFR Expression Levels of Respective Tissues and Are Responsive to EGFR-Targeted Photodynamic Therapy. *J Clin Med*, 2019, 8(11), 1880.

Fang, CY; Chen, PY; Dennis Chun-Yu Ho, Lo-Lin Tsai, Pei-Ling Hsieh, Ming-Yi Lu, Cheng-Chia Yu, Chuan-Hang Yu. miR-145 mediates the anti-cancer stemness effect of photodynamic therapy with 5-aminolevulinic acid (ALA) in oral cancer cells. *J Formos Med Assoc*, 2018, 117(8), 738-742.

Farrakhova, D; Shiryaev, A; Yakovlev, D; Efendiev, K; Maklygina, Y; Borodkin, A; Loschenov, M; Bezdetnay, L; Ryabova, A; Amirkhanova, L; Samoylova, S; Rusakov, M; Zavodnov, V; Levkin, V; Reshetov, I; Loschenov, V. Trials of a Fluorescent Endoscopic Video System for Diagnosis and Treatment of the Head and Neck Cancer. *J Clin Med*, 2019, 8(12), 2229.

Figueira, JA; Veltrini, VC. Photodynamic therapy in oral potentially malignant disorders-Critical literature review of existing protocols. *Photodiagnosis Photodyn Ther*, 2017, 20, 125-129.

Gan, J; Li, S; Meng, Y; Liao, Y; Jiang, M; Qi, L; Li, Y; Bai, Y. The influence of photodynamic therapy on the Warburg effect in esophageal cancer cells. *Lasers Med Sci*, 2020, 35(8), 1741-1750.

Ghodasra, DH; Demirci, H. Photodynamic Therapy for Choroidal Metastasis. *Am J Ophthalmol*, 2016, 161, 104-9.e1-2.

Gondivkar, SM; Gadbail, AR; Choudhary, MG; Vedpathak, PR; Likhitkar, MS. Photodynamic treatment outcomes of potentially-malignant lesions and malignancies of the head and neck region: A systematic review. *J Investig Clin Dent*, 2018, 9(1).

Grandi, V; Sessa, M; Pisano, L; Rossi, R; Galvan, A; Gattai, R; Mori, M; Tiradritti, L; Bacci, S; Zuccati, G; Cappugi, P; Pimpinelli, N. Photodynamic therapy with topical photosensitizers in mucosal and semimucosal areas: Review from a dermatologic perspective. *Photodiagnosis Photodyn Ther*, 2018, 23, 119-131.

Hosokawa, S; Takebayashi, S; Takahashi, G; Okamura, J; Mineta, H. Photodynamic therapy in patients with head and neck squamous cell carcinoma. *Lasers Surg Med*, 2018, 50(5), 420-426.

Ikeda, H; Ohba, S; Egashira, K; Asahina, I. The effect of photodynamic therapy with talaporfin sodium, a second-generation photosensitizer, on oral squamous cell carcinoma: A series of eight cases. *Photodiagnosis Photodyn Ther*, 2018, 21, 176-180.

Jerjes, W; Hamdoon, Z; Abdulkareem, AA; Hopper, C. Photodynamic therapy in the management of actinic keratosis: Retrospective evaluation of outcome. *Photodiagnosis Photodyn Ther*, 2017, 17, 200-204.

Jerjes, W; Hamdoon, Z; Hopper, C. Photodynamic therapy in the management of basal cell carcinoma: Retrospective evaluation of outcome. *Photodiagnosis Photodyn Ther*, 2017, 19, 22-27.

Jin, X; Xu, H; Deng, J; Dan, H; Ji, P; Chen, Q; Zeng, X. Photodynamic therapy for oral potentially malignant disorders. *Photodiagnosis Photodyn Ther*, 2019, 28, 146-152.

Kavuru, MS; Mehta, AC; Eliachar, I. Effect of photodynamic therapy and external beam radiation therapy on juvenile laryngotracheobronchial papillomatosis. *Am Rev Respir Dis*, 1990, 141(2), 509-10.

Kessel, D; Cho, WJ; Rakowski, J; Kim, HE; Kim, HRC. *Photochem Photobiol*, 2020, 96(3), 652-657.

Kessels, J; Hendriks, J; Nelemans, P; Mosterd, K; Kelleners-Smeets, N. Two-fold illumination in topical 5-aminolevulinic acid (ALA)-mediated photodynamic therapy (PDT) for superficial basal cell carcinoma (sBCC): A retrospective case series and cohort study. *J Am Acad Dermatol*, 2016, 74(5), 899-906.

Khachemoune, A; Barkoe, D; Braun, 3rd, M; Davison, SP. Dermatofibrosarcoma protuberans of the forehead and scalp with involvement of the outer calvarial plate: multistaged repair with the use of skin expanders. *Dermatol Surg*, 2005, 31(1), 115-9.

Kim, H; Kim, SW; Seok, KH; Hwang, CW; Ahn, JC; Jin, JO; Kang, HW. Hypericin-assisted photodynamic therapy against anaplastic thyroid cancer. *Photodiagnosis Photodyn Ther*, 2018, 24, 15-21.

Kim, J; Lim, H; Kim, S; Cho, H; Kim, Y; Li, X; Choi, H; Kim, O. Effects of HSP27 downregulation on PDT resistance through PDT-induced autophagy in head and neck cancer cells. *Oncol Rep*, 2016, 35(4), 2237-45.

Kim, SA; Lee, MR; Yoon, JH; Ahn, SQ. HOXC6 regulates the antitumor effects of pheophorbide a-based photodynamic therapy in multidrug-resistant oral cancer cells. *Int J Oncol*, 2016, 49(6), 2421-2430.

Knipping, S; Schmidt, A; Bartel-Friedrich, S. [Dilatational Tracheotomy in Head and Neck Surgery]. *Laryngorhinootologie*, 2016, 95(1), 29-36.

Kofler, B; Romani, A; Pritz, C; Steinbichler, TB; Schartinger, VH; Riechelmann, H; Dudas, J. Photodynamic Effect of Methylene Blue and Low Level Laser Radiation in Head and Neck Squamous Cell Carcinoma Cell Lines. *Int J Mol Sci*, 2018, 19(4), 1107.

Korbelik, M; Banáth, J; Zhang, W; Gallagher, P; Hode, T; Lam, S. SK; Chen, WR. N-dihydrogalactochitosan as immune and direct antitumor agent amplifying the effects of photodynamic therapy and photodynamic therapy-generated vaccines. *Int Immunopharmacol*, 2019, 75, 105764.

Korbelik, M; Banáth, J; Zhang, W; Saw, KM; Szulc, ZM; Bielawska, A; Separovic, D. Interaction of acid ceramidase inhibitor LCL521 with tumor response to photodynamic therapy and photodynamic therapy-generated vaccine. *nt J Cancer*, 2016, 139(6), 1372-8.

Kweon, S; Seok Koo, B; Jee, S. Change of Swallowing in Patients With Head and Neck Cancer After Concurrent Chemoradiotherapy. *Ann Rehabil Med*, 2016, 40(6), 1100-1107.

Lange, C; Bednarski, PJ. Evaluation for Synergistic Effects by Combinations of Photodynamic Therapy (PDT) with Temoporfin (mTHPC) and Pt(II) Complexes Carboplatin, Cisplatin or Oxaliplatin in a Set of Five Human Cancer Cell Lines. *Int J Mol Sci*, 2018, 19(10), 3183.

Lange, C; Lehmann, C; Mahler, M; Bednarski, PJ. Comparison of Cellular Death Pathways after mTHPC-mediated Photodynamic Therapy (PDT) in Five Human Cancer Cell Lines. *Cancers* (Basel), 2019, 11(5), 702.

Lecaros, RLG; Huang, L; Lee, TC; Hsu, YC. Nanoparticle Delivered VEGF-A siRNA Enhances Photodynamic Therapy for Head and Neck Cancer Treatment. *Mol Ther*, 2016, 24(1), 106-16.

Li, JW; Wu, ZM; Magetic, D; Zhang, LJ; Chen, ZL. Antitumor effects evaluation of a novel porphyrin derivative in photodynamic therapy. *Tumour Biol*, 2015, 36(12), 9685-92.

Li, X; Zhou, F; Gu, Y. Photomedicine Lights Up the Future of Fighting Cancer. *Technol Cancer Res Treat*, 2018, 18, 1-2.

Li, Y; Sui, H; Jiang, C; Li, S; Han, Y; Huang, P; Du, X; Du, J; Bai, Y. Dihydroartemisinin Increases the Sensitivity of Photodynamic Therapy Via NF-κB/HIF-1α/VEGF Pathway in Esophageal Cancer Cell *in vitro* and *in vivo*. *Cell Physiol Biochem*, 2018, 48(5), 2035-2045.

Li, Y; Wang, B; Zheng, S; He, Y. Photodynamic therapy in the treatment of oral leukoplakia: A systematic review. *Photodiagnosis Photodyn Ther*, 2019, 25, 17-22.

Liang, F; Han, P; Chen, R; Lin, P; Luo, M; Cai, Q; Huang, X. Topical 5-aminolevulinic acid photodynamic therapy for laryngeal papillomatosistosis treatment. *Photodiagnosis Photodyn Ther*, 2019, 28, 136-141.

Liu, D; Wu, L; Li, J; Shi, Li, F; Su, J; Huang, K; Zhou, Q; Zhao, S; Chen, M. Simple shaving combined with photodynamic therapy for refractory bowen disease. *Photodiagnosis Photodyn Ther*, 2019, 26, 258-260.

Liu, H; Daly, L; Rudd, G; Khan, AP; Mallidi, S; Liu, Y; Cuckov, F; Hasan, T; Celli, JP. Development and evaluation of a low-cost, portable, LED-based device for PDT treatment of early-stage oral cancer in resource-limited settings. *Lasers Surg Med*, 2019, 51(4), 345-351.

Liu, Y; Scrivano, L; Peterson, JD; Fens, M; Hernández, IB; Mesquita, B; Toraño, JS; Hennink, WE; van Nostrum, CF; Oliveira, S. EGFR-Targeted Nanobody Functionalized Polymeric Micelles Loaded with mTHPC for Selective Photodynamic Therapy. *ol Pharm*, 2020, 17(4), 1276-1292.

Liu, YQ; Meng, PS; Zhang, HC; Liu, X; Wang, MX; Cao, WW; Hu, Z; Zhang, ZG. Inhibitory effect of aloe emodin mediated photodynamic therapy on human oral mucosa carcinoma *in vitro* and *in vivo*. *Biomed Pharmacother*, 2018, 97, 697-707.

Lucky, SS; Idris, NM; Huang, K; Kim, J; Li, Z; Thong, PSP; Xu, R; Soo, KC; Zhang, Y. *In vivo* Biocompatibility, Biodistribution and Therapeutic Efficiency of Titania Coated Upconversion Nanoparticles for Photodynamic Therapy of Solid Oral Cancers. *Theranostics*, 2016, 6(11), 1844-65.

Mallidi, S; Khan, AP; Liu, H; Daly, L; Rudd, G; Leon, P; Khan, S; Hussain, BMA; Hasan, SA; Siddique, SA; Akhtar, K; August, M; Troulis, M; Cuckov, F; Celli, JP; Hasan, T. Platform for ergonomic intraoral photodynamic therapy using low-cost, modular 3D-printed components: Design, comfort and clinical evaluation. *Sci Rep*, 2019, 9(1), 15830.

Mansoori, B; Mohammadı, A; Doustvandi, MA; Mohammadnejad, F; Kamari, F; Gjerstorff, MF; Baradaran, B; Hamblin, MR. Photodynamictherapy for cancer: Role of natural products. *Photodiagnosis Photodyn Ther*, 2019, 26, 395-404.

Mao, C; Zhao, Y; Li, F; Li, Z; Tian, S; Debinski, W; Ming. XP-glycoprotein targeted and near-infrared light-guided depletion of chemoresistant tumors. *J Control Release*, 2018, 286, 289-300.

Mao, W; Sun, Y; Zhang, H; Cao, L; Wang, J; He, P. A combined modality of carboplatin and photodynamic therapy suppresses epithelial-mesenchymal transition and matrix metalloproteinase-2 (MMP-2)/MMP-9 expression in HEp-2 human laryngeal cancer cells via ROS-mediated inhibition of MEK/ERK signalling pathway. *Lasers Med Sci*, 2016, 31(8), 1697-1705.

Marchal, S; Dolivet, G; Lassalle, HP; Guillemin, F; Bezdetnaya, L. Targeted photodynamic therapy in head and neck squamous cell carcinoma: heading into the future. *Lasers Med Sci*, 2015, 30(9), 2381-7.

Meulemans, J; Delaere, P; Poorten, VV. Photodynamic therapy in head and neck cancer: indications, outcomes, and future prospects. *Curr Opin Otolaryngol Head Neck Surg*, 2019, 27(2), 136-141.

Mimikos, C; Shafirstein, G; Arshad, H. Current state and future of photodynamic therapy for the treatment of head and neck squamous cell carcinoma. *World J Otorhinolaryngol Head Neck Surg*, 2016, 2(2), 126-129.

Minamide, T; Yoda, Y; Hori, K; Shinmura, K; Oono, Y; Ikematsu, H; Yano, T. Advantages of salvage photodynamic therapy using talaporfin sodium for local failure after chemoradiotherapy or radiotherapy for esophageal cancer. *Surg Endosc*, 2020, 34(2), 899-906.

Muhanna, N; Chan, HHL; Townson, JT; Jin, CS; Ding, L; Valic, M. S; Douglas, CM; MacLaughlin, CM; Chen, J; Zheng, G; Irish, JC. Photodynamic therapy enables tumor-specific ablation in preclinical models of thyroid cancer. *Endocr Relat Cancer*, 2020, 27(2), 41-53.

Muhanna, N; Cui, L; Chan, H; Burgess, L; Jin, CS; MacDonald, T. D; Huynh, E; Wang, F; Chen, J; Irish, JC; Zheng, G. Multimodal Image-Guided Surgical and Photodynamic Interventions in Head and Neck Cancer: From Primary Tumor to Metastatic Drainage. *Clin Cancer Res*, 2016, 22(4), 961-70.

Nishie, H; Kataoka, H; Yano, S; Kikuchi, JI; Hayashi, N; Narumi, A; Nomoto, A; Kubota, E; Joh, T. A next-generation bifunctional photosensitizer with improved water-solubility for photodynamic therapy and diagnosis. *Oncotarget*, 2016, 7(45), 74259-74268.

Oakley, E; Bellnier, DA; Hutson, A; Wrazen, B; Arshad, H; Quon, H; Shafirstein, G. Surface markers for guiding cylindrical diffuser fiber insertion in interstitial photodynamic therapy of head and neck cancer. *Lasers Surg Med*, 2017, 49(6), 599-608.

Obstoy, B; Salaun, M; Bohn, P; Veresezan, L; Sesboué, R; Thiberville, L. Photodynamic therapy using methylene blue in lung adenocarcinoma xenograft and hamster cheek pouch induced squamous cell carcinoma. *Photodiagnosis Photodyn Ther*, 2016, 15, 109-14.

Palumbo, MN; Cervantes, O; Eugênio, C; Hortense, FTP; Ribeiro, JC; Paolini, AAP; Tedesco, AC; Sercarz, JA; Paiva, M. B. Intratumor cisplatin nephrotoxicity in combined laser-induced thermal therapy for cancer treatment. *Lasers Surg Med*, 2017, 49(8), 756-762.

Peng, W; de Bruijn, HS; Ten Hagen, TLM; van Dam, GM; Roodenburg, JLN; Berg, K; Witjes, MJH; Robinson, DJ. Targeted Photodynamic Therapy of Human Head and Neck Squamous Cell Carcinoma with Anti-epidermal Growth Factor Receptor Antibody Cetuximab and Photosensitizer IR700DX in the Mouse Skin-fold Window Chamber Model. *Photochem Photobiol*, 2020, 96(3), 708-717.

Pfefer, TJ; Schomacker, KT; Nishioka, NS. Long-term effects of photodynamic therapy on fluorescence spectroscopy in the human esophagus. *Photochem Photobiol*, 2001.

Pfefer, TJ; Schomacker, KT; Nishioka, NS. Long-term effects of photo dynamic therapy on fluorescence spectroscopy in the humanesophagus. *Photochem Photobiol*, 2001, 73(6), 664-8.

Pramual, S; Lirdprapamongkol, K; Svasti, J; Bergkvist, M; Jouan-Hureaux, V; Arnoux, P; Frochot, C; Barberi-Heyob, M; Niamsiri, N. Polymer-lipid-PEG hybrid nanoparticles as photosensitizer carrier for photodynamic therapy. *J Photochem Photobiol B*, 2017, 173, 12-22.

Qiao, L; Mei, Z; Yang, Z; Li, X; Cai, H; Liu, W. ALA-PDT inhibits proliferation and promotes apoptosis of SCC cells through STAT3 signal pathway. *Photodiagnosis Photodyn Ther*, 2016, 14, 66-73.

Quintanilha, NP; Irina Dos Santos Miranda Costa 1, de Souza Ramos, MF; de Miguel, NCO; Pierre, MBR. α-Bisabolol improves 5-aminolevulinic acid retention in buccal tissues: Potential application in the photodynamic therapy of oral cancer. *J Photochem Photobiol B*, 2017, 174, 298-305.

Ren, S; Cheng, X; Chen, M; Liu, C; Zhao, P; Huang, W; He, J; Zhou, Z; Miao, L. Hypotoxic and Rapidly Metabolic PEG-PCL-C3-ICG Nanoparticles for Fluorescence-Guided Photothermal/Photodynamic Therapy against OSCC. *ACS Appl Mater Interfaces*, 2017, 9(37), 31509-31518.

Rohrbach, DJ; Rigual, N; Arshad, H; Tracy, EC; Cooper, MT; Shafirstein, G; Wilding, G; Merzianu, M; Baumann, H; Henderson, BW; Sunar, U. Intraoperative optical assessment of photodynamic therapy response of superficial oral squamous cell carcinoma. *J Biomed Opt*, 2016, 21(1), 18002.

Rosin, FCP; Teixeira, MG; Pelissari, C; Corrêa, L. Photodynamic Therapy Mediated by 5-aminolevulinic Acid Promotes the Upregulation and Modifies the Intracellular Expression of Surveillance Proteins in Oral Squamous Cell Carcinoma. *Photochem Photobiol*, 2019, 95(2), 635-643.

Rosin, FCP; Teixeira, MG; Pelissari, C; Corrêa, L. Resistance of oral cancer cells to 5-ALA-mediated photodynamic therapy. *J Cell Biochem*, 2018, 119(4), 3554-3562.

Santos, LL; Oliveira, J; Monteiro, E; Santos, J; Sarmento, C. Treatment of Head and Neck Cancer with Photodynamic Therapy with Redaporfin: A Clinical Case Report. *Case Rep Oncol*, 2018 Nov, 11(3), 769-776.

Shafirstein, G; Bellnier, D; Oakley, E; Hamilton, S; Potasek, M; Beeson, K; Parilov, E. Interstitial Photodynamic Therapy-A Focused Review. *Cancers* (Basel), 2017, 9(2), 12.

Shafirstein, G; Bellnier, DA; Oakley, E; Hamilton, S; Habitzruther, M; Tworek, L; Hutson, A; Spernyak, JA; Sexton, S; Curtin, L; Turowski, SG; Arshad, H; Henderson, B. Irradiance controls photodynamic efficacy and tissue heating in experimental tumours: implication for interstitial PDT of locally advanced cancer. *Br J Cancer*, 2018, 119(10), 1191-1199.

Shafirstein, G; Rigual, NR; Arshad, H; Cooper, MT; Bellnier, DA; Wilding, G; Tan, W; Merzianu, M; Henderson, BW. Photodynamic therapy with 3-(1'-hexyloxyethyl) pyropheophorbide-a for early-stage cancer of the larynx: Phase Ib study. *Head Neck*, 2016, 38 Suppl 1(Suppl 1), E377-83.

Shen, L; Huang, Y; Chen, D; Qiu, F; Ma, C; Jin, X; Zhu, X; Zhou, G; Zhang, Z. pH-Responsive Aerobic Nanoparticles for Effective Photodynamic Therapy. *Theranostics*, 2017, 7(18), 4537-4550.

Shi, R; Li, C; Jiang, Z; Li, W; Wang, A; Wei, J. Preclinical Study of Antineoplastic Sinoporphyrin Sodium-PDT via *In Vitro* and *In Vivo* Models. *Molecules*, 2017, 22(1), 112.

Shi, S; Cho, H; Sun, Q; He, Y; Ma, G; Kim, Y; Kim, B; Kim, O. Acanthopanacis Cortex extract: A novel photosensitizer for head and neck squamous cell carcinoma therapy. *Photodiagnosis Photodyn Ther; Photodiagnosis Photodyn Ther*, 2019, 26, 142-149.

Shi, Y; Zhang, B; Feng, X; Qu, F; Wang, S; Wu, L; Wang, X; Liu, Q; Wang, P; Zhang, K. Apoptosis and autophagy induced by DVDMs-PDT on human esophageal cancer Eca-109 cells. *Photodiagnosis Photodyn Ther*, 2018, 24, 198-205.

Sotiriou, E; Apalla, Z; Vrani, F; Lazaridou, E; Vakirlis, E; Lallas, A; Ioannides, D. Daylight photodynamic therapy vs. Conventional photodynamic therapy as skin cancer preventive treatment in patients with face and scalp cancerization: an intra-individual comparison study. *J Eur Acad Dermatol Venereol*, 2017, 31(8), 1 303-1307.

Theodoraki, MN; Lorenz, K; Lotfi, R; Fürst, D; Tsamadou, C; Jaekle, S; Mytilineos, J; Brunner, C; Theodorakis, J; Hoffmann, TK; Laban, S; Schuler, PJ. Influence of photodynamic therapy on peripheral immune cell populations and cytokine concentrations in head and neck cancer. *Photodiagnosis Photodyn Ther*, 2017, 19, 194-201.

Theodoraki, MN; Lorenz, KJ; Schneider, J; Thierauf, JC; Spagnoli, G; Schuler, PJ; Hoffmann, TK; Laban, S. Influence of Photodynamic Therapy on the Expression of Cancer/Testis Antigens in Squamous Cell Carcinoma of the Head and Neck. *Anticancer Res*, 2016, 36(8), 3973-82.

Theodoraki, MN; Yerneni, SS; Brunner, C; Theodorakis, J; Hoffmann, TK; Whiteside, TL. Plasma-derived Exosomes Reverse Epithelial-to-Mesenchymal Transition after Photodynamic Therapy of Patients with Head and Neck Cancer. *Oncoscience*, 2018, 5(3-4), 75-87.

Tsunoi, Y; Araki, K; Ozeki, E; Hara, I; Shiotani, A; Terakawa, M; Sato, S. Photoacoustic diagnosis of pharmacokinetics and vascular shutdown effects in photodynamic treatment with indocyanine green-lactosome for a subcutaneous tumor in mice. *Photodiagnosis Photodyn Ther*, 2019, 26, 436-441.

van Doeveren, TEM; Karakullukçu, MB; van Veen, RLP; Lopez-Yurda, M; Schreuder, WH; Tan, IB. Adjuvant photodynamic therapy in head and neck cancer after tumor-positive resection margins. *Laryngoscope*, 2018, 128(3), 657-663.

van Driel, PBAA; Boonstra, MC; Slooter, MD; Heukers, R; Stammes, MA; Snoeks, TJA; de Bruijn, HS; van Diest, PJ; Vahrmeijer, AL; van Bergen En Henegouwen, PMP; van de Velde, CJH; Löwik, CWGM; Robinson, DJ; Oliveira, S. EGFR targeted nanobody-photosensitizer conjugates for photodynamic therapy in a pre-clinical model of head and neck cancer. *J Control Release*, 2016, 229, 93-105.

van Straten, D; Mashayekhi, V; de Bruijn, HS; Oliveira, S; Robinson, DJ. Oncologic Photodynamic Therapy: Basic Principles, Current Clinical Status and Future Directions. *Cancers* (Basel), 2017, 9(2), 19.

Volgger, V; Betz, CS. Photodynamic therapy in the upper aerodigestive tract. Overview and outlook. *J Biophotonics*, 2016, 9(11-12), 1302-1313.

Vrani, F; Sotiriou, E; Lazaridou, E; Vakirlis, E; Sideris, N; Kirmanidou, E; Apalla, Z; Lallas, A; Ioannides, D. Short incubation fractional CO_2 laser-assisted photodynamic therapy vs. conventional photodynamic therapy in field-cancerized skin: 12-month follow-up results of a randomized intraindividual comparison study. *J Eur Acad Dermatol Venereol*, 2019, 33(1), 79-83.

Wang, J; Liu, Q; Zhang, Y; Shi, H; Liu, H; Guo, W; Ma, Y; Huang, W; Hong, Z. Folic Acid-Conjugated Pyropheophorbide a as the Photosensitizer Tested for *In Vivo* Targeted Photodynamic *Therapy. J Pharm Sci*, 2017, 106(6), 1482-1489.

Wang, Y; Xie, D; Pan, J; Xia, C; Fan, L; Pu, Y; Zhang, Q; Ni, Y. H; Wang, J; Hu, Q. A near infrared light-triggered human serum albumin drug delivery system with coordination bonding of indocyanine green and cisplatin for targeting photochemistry therapy against oral squamous cell cancer. *Biomater Sci*, 2019, 7(12), 5270-5282.

Wu, H; Minamide, T; Yano, T. Role of photodynamic therapy in the treatment of esophageal cancer, *Dig Endosc*, 2019, 31(5), 508-516.

Xian, W; Duleba, M; Zhang, Y; Yamamoto, Y; Ho, KY; Crum, C; McKeon, F. The Cellular Origin of Barrett's Esophagus and Its Stem Cells. *Adv Exp Med Biol*, 2019, 1123, 55-69.

Xiao, J; Cheng, L; Fang, T; Zhang, Y; Zhou, J; Cheng, R; Tang, W; Zhong, X; Lu, Y; Deng, L; Cheng, Y; Zhu, Y; Liu, Z; Cui, W. Nanoparticle-Embedded Electrospun Fiber-Covered Stent to Assist Intraluminal Photodynamic Treatment of Oesophageal Cancer. *Small*, 2019, 15(49), e1904979.

Xue, K; Wang, YN; Zhao, X; Zhang, HX; Yu, D; Jin, CS. Synergistic effect of meta-tetra(hydroxyphenyl)chlorin-based photodynamic therapy followed by cisplatin on malignant Hep-2 cells. *Onco Targets Ther*, 2019, 12, 5525-5536.

Yachimski, P; Puricelli, WP; Nishioka, NS. *Patient predictors of esophageal stricture development after photodynamic therapy*, 2008, 6(3), 302-8.

Yang, PW; Chiang, TH; Hsieh, CY; Huang, YC; Wong, LF; Hung, MC; Tsai, JC; Lee, JM. The effect of ephrin-A1 on resistance to Photofrin-mediated photodynamic therapy in esophageal squamous cell carcinoma cells. *Lasers Med Sci*, 2015, 30(9), 2353-61.

Yang, Y; Tu, J; Yang, D; Raymond, JL; Roy, RA; Zhang, D. Photo- and Sono-Dynamic Therapy: A Review of Mechanisms and Considerations for Pharmacological Agents Used in Therapy Incorporating Light and Sound. *Curr Pharm Des*, 2019, 25(4), 401-412.

Yanovsky, RL; Bartenstein, DW; Rogers, GS; Isakoff, SJ; Chen, ST. Photodynamic therapy for solid tumors: A review of the literature. *Photodermatol Photoimmunol Photomed*, 2019, 35(5), 295-303.

Zecha, JAEM; Raber- Durlacher, E; Nair, RG; Epstein, JB; Sonis, S. T; Elad, S; Hamblin, MR; Barasch, A; Migliorati, CA; Milstein, D. MJ; Genot, MT; Lansaat, L; van der Brink, R; Arnabat-Dominguez, J; van der Molen, L; Jacobi, I; van Diessen, J; de Lange, J; Smeele, LE; Schubert, MM; Bensadoun, RJ. Low level laser therapy/ photobiomodulation in the management of side effects of chemoradiation therapy in head and neck cancer: part 1: mechanisms of action, dosimetric, and safety considerations. *Support Care Cancer*, 2016, 24(6), 2781-92.

Zecha, JAEM; Raber- Durlacher, JE; Nair, RG; Epstein, JB; Elad, S; Hamblin, MR; Barasch, A; Migliorati, CA; Milstein, DMJ; Genot, MT; Lansaat, L; van der Brink, R; Arnabat-Dominguez, J; van der Molen, L; Jacobi, I; van Diessen, J; de Lange, J; Smeele, LE; Schubert, MM; Bensadoun, RJ. *Low-level laser therapy/photobiomodulation in the management of side effects of chemoradiation therapy in head and neck cancer: part 2: proposed applications and treatment protocols Support Care Cancer*, 2016, 24(6), 2793-805.

Zhang, C; Jiang, JQ. [Current status and prospect of photodynamic therapy in laryngeal diseases]. *Zhonghua Er Bi Yan Hou Tou Jing Wai Ke Za Zhi*, 2018, 53(4), 306-311.

Zhang, CY; Zhang, LJ; Li, JW; Li, JH; Wu, ZM; Zhang, LX; Chen, N; Yan, YJ; Chen, ZL. *In vitro* and *in vivo* antitumor activity of a novel chlorin derivative for photodynamic therapy. *Neoplasma*, 2016, 63(1), 37-43.

Zhu, T; Shi, L; Yu, C; Dong, Y; Qiu, F; Shen, L; Qian, Q; Zhou, G; Zhu, X. Ferroptosis Promotes Photodynamic Therapy: Supramolecular Photosensitizer-Inducer Nanodrug for Enhanced Cancer Treatment. *Theranostics*, 2019, 9(11), 3293-3307.

Chapter 6

THE USE OF LASER LIGHT IN LARYNGOLOGY

Wojciech Domka, David Aebisher, Lidia Bieniasz and Dorota Bartusik-Aebisher[*]
Medical College of The University of Rzeszów

ABSTRACT

Photodynamic therapy (PDT) for squamous cell carcinoma of the head and neck is an established anti-cancer therapy that, by combining a photosensitizing agent (PS) with light and oxygen. PDT produces highly cytotoxic reactive oxygen species, leading to selective tumor eradication. Improving tumor selectivity is a major challenge that can be addressed by using a new generation of photosensitizing nanoparticles.

Keywords: photodynamic effect, therapy, cancer

Photodynamic Therapy (PDT) offers a therapeutic solution that has been found to be cost-effective compared to palliative major surgery or

---

[*] Corresponding Author's Email: dbartusik-aebisher@ur.edu.pl.

chemotherapy. However, despite the significant improvement noted in preclinical and clinical trials, PDT is still not considered the standard treatment option for head and neck cancer (Zecha et al., 2016; Strand et al., 2017; Krowchuk et al., 2019; Whelan. et al., 2019; Klimza et al., 2019; Mosca et al., 2019; Jain et al., 2016; Dehkordi et al., 2015; Lou et al., 2019). PDT can eliminate tumors that are resistant to chemoradiotherapy strategies - again, an all too common problem with recurrent cases of head and neck cancer. In otolaryngology, CO_2 laser is the first and most commonly applied device. Such lasers as Ny:YAG generating visible light having wavelength 532 nm referred to as KTP laser due to the (Wojdas, et al., 2009; Augustin et al., 2010; Buckmiller et al., 2010; Eckert et al., 2011; Macheda et al., 2005; Nonoga et al., 2010; Renkonen et al., 2013; Zhang et al., 2010; Gronkiewicz et al., 2014; Swartz et al., 2015; Swartz et al., 2015; Biesaga et al., 2008; Song et al., 2006; Tirakotai et al., 2006; Hélen et al., 2014). PDT treatments offer substantial advantages over radiotherapy as well as chemoradiation treatments. Moreover, PDT can eliminate tumors that are resistant to chemoradiation strategies. But for those patients who are considered to be unsuitable for the therapeutic options listed above, PDT can be offered as a reasonable and effective treatment option. At this point, PDT appears to be particularly efficient in treating cancers of the mouth and throat. Porphyrins are a group of substances that serve as some of the most potent photosensitizers in the realm of photomedicine. PDT is an attractive treatment for focal therapy of localized tumors, especially in the case of unresectable tumors (Marchal et al., 2015; Wojdas et al., 2009; Atkins et al., 1984; Marchal et al., 2015; Boppana et al., 2015; Chen et al., 2015; He et al., 2015; Lu et al., 2014; Lee et al., 2015; Argiris et al., 2008; Hang Yang 2019; Zhou et al., 2017; Wei et al., 2018; Marius et al., 2016; Chen-Xi et al., 2016; Kehinde et al., 2012). In addition, some photosensitizers hold high fluorescence yield and therefore could emerge as theranostic agents (Marchal et al., 2015). Head and neck cancers include a heterogeneous group of tumors involving the oral cavity, pharynx, larynx, nasal and sinus cavities, orbit, and other related structures like the skin. PDT therapy is an established anticancer treatment that requires a photosensitizer which accumulates preferentially in malignant tissue, nonthermal visible light and molecular oxygen. PDT is still not considered as a standard treatment option of head and neck cancers. Combining PDT with another anticancer treatment modality is an important strategy for improved efficacy (Boppana et al., 2015). Combination therapy has become a major strategy in cancer treatment (Chena et al., 2015). The study suggests multifunctional core-shell nanoparticles as a versatile and effective drug delivery system for potential translation to the clinic (He et al., 2015). PDT is an effective anticancer procedure that relies on tumor localization of a photosensitizer followed by light activation to generate cytotoxic reactive oxygen species (e.g., $^1O_2$) (Lu et al., 2014; Lee et al., 2015). PDT is a method to treat cancers using photosensitizer and light. PDT has been tried already for several tumors. However, the clinical applications are limited by the toxicity of photosensitizer and narrow effect. Cell viability was decreased significantly by combination treatment (Argiris et al., 2008; Yang et al., 2019; Zhou et al., 2017; Wei et al., 2018; Marius et al., 2016; Chen-Xi et al., 2016; Adekola et al., 2012; Augustin et al., 2010; Buckmiller et al., 2010; Eckert et al., 2011; Macheda et al., 2005; Suel et al., 2010; Renkonen et al., 2013; Zhang et al., 2010; Gronkiewicz et al., 2014; Swartz et al., 2015; Biesaga et al., 2008; Song et al., 2006; Tirakotai 2006; Denise 2014). With regard to rates of mortality, intraoperative hemorrhage, and postoperative hemorrhage, there was no statistically significant difference between the two techniques.: In critically ill patients, PDT appears to be a safe alternative (Yang et al., 2019). PDT is a clinically approved cancer therapy, based on a photochemical reaction between a light activatable molecule or photosensitizer, light, and molecular oxygen. PDT is a two-stage procedure, which starts with photosensitizer administration followed by a locally directed light exposure, with the aim of confined tumor destruction (Civantos et al., 2018). PDT involves the use of a phototoxic drug which is activated by low powered laser light to destroy neoplastic cells. Multiple photosensitizers have been studied and tumors have been treated in a variety of head and neck sites over the last 30 years (Civantos et al., 2018). Detection reactive oxygen species and mitochondrial membrane potential after HYP-assisted PDT were analyzed by confocal microscopy (Kim et al., 2018). Photodynamic therapy is a promising treatment modality for laryngeal dysplasia, early-stage carcinoma, and papilloma, and was reported to have the ability to preserve laryngeal function and voice quality without clinical fibrotic response (Zhang et al., 2018). Cell viability in response to varying doses of PDT was investigated by the Cell Counting Kit-8 method (Zhang et al., 2018). PDT may be useful in treating existing vocal fold scars. Further studies should focus on the *in vivo* effect of PDT on vocal fold wound healing and scar remodeling (Volgger et al., 2016). Nevertheless, further clinical studies are needed to better define its true value in head and neck oncology (Tsunoi et al., 2019). Indocyanine green lactosome is an attractive new-generation agent for photodynamic therapy that is characterized by a near-infrared excitation wavelength and high stability in the bloodstream (Cerrati et al., 2015). Photodynamic therapy is a palliative treatment option for head and neck squamous cell carcinoma patients which induces local inflammation and alters tumor cell morphology (Theodoraki et al., 2018). Fiberoptic tracheo-bronchoscopy is the most commonly used procedure for percutaneous dilational tracheotomy (Nowak et al., 2017). PDT is possible (Nowak et al., 2017). PDT is a relatively new alternative method of performing PDTs in which tissues overlying the trachea are dissected, but needle entry is still performed blindly (Gadkaree et al., 2016). Percutaneous dilational tracheostomy can be performed with similarly low complication rates with or without the use of bronchoscopy. Discontinuing the use of bronchoscopy in these procedures appears to be a safe, cost-effective alternative with reassuring outcomes and low complication rates. The high expense and logistical barriers to obtaining treatment with surgery, radiotherapy and chemotherapy often result in progression to unmanageable late stage disease with high morbidity (Mallidi et al., 2019). PDT using BF-200 ALA has recently been clinically approved and is under investigation in several phase III trials for the treatment of actinic keratosis. This study is the first to compare BF-200 ALA with ALA in preclinical models (de Bruijn et al., 2016). The present study illustrates the clinical potential of light fractionated PDT using BF-200 ALA for enhancing PDT efficacy in (pre-) malignant skin conditions such as basal cell carcinoma and vulval intraepithelial neoplasia and its application in other lesion such as cervical intraepithelial neoplasia and oral squamous cell carcinoma where current approaches have limited efficacy (de Bruijn et al., 2016). The incidence of differentiated thyroid cancer has increased significantly during the last several decades. Photodynamic therapy has the potential to reduce treatment-related side effects by decreasing invasiveness and limiting toxicity (Muhanna et al., 2020). This resulted in significant and specific apoptosis in tumor tissue, but not surrounding normal tissues including trachea and recurrent laryngeal nerve (Muhanna et al., 2020). Conclusion: GWB-PDT is a feasible and safe solution for tracheostomies in general-ward ventilated patients (Cohen et al., 2018). To evaluate the feasibility of topical photodynamic therapy using 5-aminolevulinic acid (5-ALA) for vocal fold leukoplakia. The penetration depth and concentrations of 5-ALA in tissue were quantified using frozen sectioning and fluorescamine derivatization after 5-ALA contact incubation or topical spraying (Zhang et al., 2019). Topical PDT with laryngeal spraying of 20% 5-ALA solution achieves sufficient therapeutic effects and is potentially applicable for the treatment of vocal fold leukoplakia (Chatterjee et al., 2018). Palliative treatments like photodynamic therapy are being implemented for a long time however, the results are still not promising in case of aggressive cancers like anaplastic thyroid cancer. The objective of this work is to establish an alternative method with the combination of photofrin-PDT and sulforaphene, a natural isothiocyanate from cruciferous vegetables, against human anaplastic thyroid cancer to enhance the efficacy of PDT. PDT and SFE can induce apoptosis in anaplastic thyroid cancer cells individually but while treated in combination, it enhanced the apoptotic and anti-proliferative effect, much higher than the individual doses. In summary, our work designates sulforaphene as a unique natural enhancer of efficacy with PDT against anaplastic thyroid cancer. Different photosensitizer-mediated photodynamic therapy has different intracellular cytotoxic cascades (Wang et al., 2014). This study demonstrates that a sublethal dose of m-THPC PDT inhibits the migration and invasion of nasopharyngeal carcinoma cells *in vitro* (Wang et al., 2014). In this study the authors report on vascular responses induced by ALA-PDT for different fluence rates, including both changes in vessel diameter and dynamics in RBC velocity in arterioles, imaged using intra-vital confocal microscopy in skinfold chambers in hairless mice. Our interest is in the dynamics of vascular changes in the early stages of illumination (van Leeuwen-van Zaane et al., 2014). In this study, a significant difference between fluence rates. Arterioles were particularly sensitive to vasoconstriction during low dose PDT, often resulting in complete vasoconstriction. Since the therapeutic effects of PDT are dependent on a fine balance between the need for oxygen during illumination and disruption of the vasculature, the results of the present study add to our understanding of acute vascular effects during ALA-PDT and aid our efforts to optimize PDT using porphyrin pre-cursors (Manivasagan, et al., 2018). Numerous studies have shown that marine natural pigments have considerable medicinal potential and promising applications in human health (Manivasagan, et al., 2018). the marine natural pigments as potential sources for therapeutic applications, including: antioxidant, anticancer, antiangiogenic, anti-obesity, anti-inflammatory activities, drug delivery, photothermal therapy, photodynamic therapy photoacoustic imaging, and wound healing. Marine natural pigments will offer a better platform for future theranostic applications (Manivasagan, et al., 2018). Recent studies have indicated that cancer stem-like cells exhibit a high resistance to current therapeutic strategies, including photodynamic therapy, leading to the recurrence and progression of colorectal cancer. In cancer, autophagy acts as both a tumor suppressor and a tumor promoter (Wei et al., 2014). Percutaneous dilatational tracheostomy has become a standard technique for critically ill patients who require long-term ventilation. The most common early post-operative complication is bleeding related to anatomical variation in vasculature. The procedure is performed at the patient's bedside unless this is deemed unsafe and then the accepted alternative is open tracheostomy in the operating room (Even-Tov et al., 2017). Following ultrasound examination, the management decision was changed in nine patients (Even-Tov et al., 2017). Pre-procedural ultrasound for critically ill patients undergoing tracheostomy can influence management decisions regarding the performance of tracheostomy (Even-Tov et al., 2017). Percutaneous dilatational tracheostomy has become a standard technique for critically ill patients who require long-term ventilation. The most common early post-operative complication is bleeding related to anatomical variation in vasculature. The procedure is performed at the patient's bedside unless this is deemed unsafe and then the accepted alternative is open tracheostomy in the operating room (Even-Tov et al., 2017). To evaluate the use of pre-procedural ultrasound to aid in the decision of whether PDT in critical care patients should be performed at the patient's bedside or by open surgical tracheostomy (Even-Tov et al., 2017). Patients were jointly evaluated by a critical care physician and a head and neck surgeon. Based on this evaluation, the method of tracheostomy was determined. Subsequently, pre-procedural ultrasound examination of the anterior neck was performed. The final decision whether to perform PDT or open surgical tracheostomy was based on the ultrasound findings. Changes in management decisions following ultrasound were recorded. Following ultrasound examination, the management decision was changed in nine patients (25Pre-procedural ultrasound for critically ill patients undergoing tracheostomy can influence management decisions regarding the performance of tracheostomy. Topical photodynamic therapy is a successful treatment for nonmelanotic skin cancers. Nevertheless, surgical excision continues to be the gold standard treatment. Cervicofaial excision often results in functional and aesthetic impairment. (Jeremic et al., 2011). To determine the utility of PDT in reducing the NMSC area for the purpose of surgical excision. Of these lesions, 22 demonstrated a complete curative response after an average of two PDT treatments, which were then confirmed with histologically negative biopsies. These lesions were then excised with clear histologic margins. Follow-up at 1 year for all lesions demonstrated no locoregional recurrence. This is the first study to investigate the efficacy of neoadjuvant topical PDT in the management of NMSC. The results suggest that for NMSC not demonstrating a complete curative response to PDT, neoadjuvant PDT can substantially reduce tumour burden, allowing for less morbid surgical excisions with histologically clear margins. To compare the ultra percutaneous dilation tracheostomy and mini open techniques in randomized fixed and fresh cadavers. Assess degrees of damage to tracheal cartilage and mucosa via tracheal lumen and external dissection (Al-Qahtani et al., 2015). . PDT resulted in severe damage to mucosa and cartilage, that might contribute to subglottic stenosis preventing decannulation. Considering the injury, MOT has better outcome than UPDT. Photodynamic therapy utilizing aminolevulinic acid (ALA) as a photosensitiser has been used to ablate premalignant/malignant skin conditions including superficial basal cell carcinoma with acceptable cosmetic outcome. Clinicians continue however to face difficulties in determining the exact dose that is sufficient to achieve a complete healing from the condition where the experience of the clinician remains the only determinant factor. This inaccuracy sometimes leads to undertreating these lesions (Sharwani et al., 2104). By comparison, the post- PDT red fluorescence values in cheek and scalp were lower than that of the temple and nose, respectively; this may be a useful indicative of the response rate of tissue to therapy. Staphylococcus aureus (S. aureus) is hard to be eradicated, not only due to the emergence of antibiotic resistant strains but also because of its ability to form biofilm. Antibiotics are the major approach to treating biofilm infections, but their effects are unsatisfactory. One of the potential alternative treatments for controlling biofilm infections is photodynamic therapy (PDT), which requires the administration of photosensitizer, followed by light activation (Zhang et al., 2017). 5-aminolevulinic acid a natural photosensitizer prodrug, presents favorable characteristics, such as easy penetration and rapid clearance. These advantages enable ALA-based PDT to be well-tolerated by patients and it can be repeatedly applied without cumulative toxicity or serious side effects. ALA-PDT has been proven to be an effective treatment for multidrug resistant pathogens; however, the study of its effect on S. aureus biofilm is limited. The results showed that ALA-PDT has a strong antibacterial effect on S. aureus biofilm, which was confirmed by the confocal laser scanning microscope. In addition, the improved bactericidal effect was observed in the combined treatment group but in a strain-dependent manner. Our results suggest that ALA-PDT is a potential alternative approach for future clinical use to treat S. aureus biofilm-associated infections, and some patients may benefit from the combined treatment of ALA-PDT and antibiotics, but drug sensitivity testing should be performed in advance. In 2009, percutaneous dilational tracheotomy (PDT) in otolaryngology residency training. PDT was performed in 21 cases and five residents had an opportunity to learn PDT. No major complications occurred. Decannulation was achieved in 17 of the 18 cases, excluding 3 mortalities. All residents felt that their knowledge of PDT had advanced. Introduction of PDT has great significance in otolaryngology residency training (Furuta et al., 2015). Photodynamic therapy is a promising treatment modality for malignant diseases through the generation of reactive oxygen species (Zhang et al., 2014). Following PDT, ROS were measured by a fluorescence microscope in both the presence and absence of glutathione (GSH) pretreatment. Wound healing assay, cell migration assay, and matrigel invasion assay were used to evaluate the cellular migration and invasion. Western blot was performed to investigate the signaling pathways that may have been involved. ROS were rapidly generated in 9-HPbD-loaded HEp-2 laryngeal cancer cells by the activation of a diode laser and were significantly inhibited by a 6 h GSH pretreatment. Wound healing assay, cell migration assay, and matrigel invasion assay showed that sublethal PDT significantly suppressed the migration and invasion of HEp-2 cells (Ahn et al., 2018). Measurement of the physiologic properties of target lesions may allow for identification of patients with the highest probability of benefiting from PDT. This provides opportunity for optimizing light delivery based on lesion characteristics and/or informing ongoing clinical decision-making in patients who would most benefit from PDT. To investigate the diffusion changes in both the optic nerve and optic tract in orbital space-occupying lesion patients with decreased visual acuity, and its clinical significance using probabilistic diffusion tractography (Wu et al., 2019). Twenty patients with orbital space-occupying lesions and 25 age- and gender-matched healthy persons were included. (Wu et al., 2019). FA, MD, AD, and RD of the affected side optic nerve of the orbital space-occupying lesions have significantly changed, the FA value is the most sensitive. The PDT could be a useful tool to provide valid quantitative markers of optic nerve injuries and evaluate the severity of orbital diseases, which other examinations cannot be acquired. Tumor drug resistance limits the response to chemotherapy. Interestingly, sequential combination therapy enhances the anticancer efficacy of drugs like cisplatin (CDDP) via synergistic effects. (Xue et al., 2019). In the cultured Hep-2 cells, meta-tetra (hydroxyphenyl)chlorin (m-THPC) and CDDP were administered separately or in combination (Xue et al., 2019). The sequential treatment significantly diminished cell viability and induced cell apoptosis, in consistency with the usage of single therapeutic strategies, as reflected by an increase in Bax expression and decrease of Bcl-2 expression. The application of sequential treatment of PDT in combination with chemotherapy offers a promising therapeutic option for cancer treatment, by regulating the PD-L1 expression, autophagy, and non-mitochondrial pathways. This article presents a review of the modern specialized medical literature concerned with the applications of photodynamic therapy (PDT) in otorhinolaryngology and medicine at large. The necessity of such a review of the available possibilities provided by PDT is dictated by the ever increasing interest of otorhinolaryngologists and specialists of other medical disciplines in the use of this method for the treatment of tumours and inflammatory diseases as well as their pyogenic complications. The author offers the critical assessment of the experience gained with the application of the known PDT technologies for the management of various pathological conditions. Especially much attention is given to the treatment of acute and chronic inflammation in the otorhinolaryngological practice with special reference to the yet unresolved problems (Lapchenko, 2015). Photodynamic therapy has been developed as a viable treatment for cancer, while apoptin is an apoptosis-inducing protein. This study was undertaken to evaluate the feasibility and efficacy of apoptin with photodynamic therapy (PDT) in the treatment of nasopharyngeal carcinoma (Fang et al., 2012). RT-PCR and western blotting were used to detect the expression of apoptin in CNE-2 NPC cells. MTT and flow cytometry analysis were used to detect cell proliferation and cell apoptosis, respectively. Transmission electron microscopy was used to observe cell structures. Hematoxylin and eosin staining was used to observe the xenograft morphology. The expression of apoptin was analyzed by RT-PCR and western blotting in CNE-2 cells stably transfected with PVP3 plasmid. Apoptin restrained cell proliferation and enhanced cell apoptosis compared to controls. He study show that apoptin in combination with PDT has a better therapeutic effect in NPC than PDT therapy or apoptin gene therapy alone (Fang et al., 2012). Photodynamic therapy represents a palliative treatment option for a selected group of patients with head and neck squamous cell carcinoma (HNSCC). PDT induces a local inflammatory reaction with the potential to initiate antitumor immune responses. However, the systemic impact on peripheral immune cells has not been described so far (Theodoraki et al., 2017). Targeted photodynamic therapy has the potential to improve the therapeutic effect of PDT due to significantly better tumor responses and less normal tissue damage (Peng et al., 2020). Cell survival after treatment with different fluence rates was investigated in three cell lines. Singlet oxygen formation was investigated using the singlet oxygen quencher sodium azide and singlet oxygen sensor green. The effectiveness of targeted PDT is, like PDT, dependent on the generation of singlet oxygen and thus the availability of intracellular oxygen (Peng et al., 2020). Fatal complications of percutaneous dilatational tracheostomy are rare and intraoperative fatal complications of PDT even more so. We present the unique case of a fatal nonvascular intraoperative complication of PDT, previously unreported in the medical literature. The authors also present a review of all previously reported fatal complications of PDT (Gilbey et al., 2012). A review of all previously reported fatal complications of PDT was conducted in order to examine the prevalent causes of death and to attempt to recommend measures designed to prevent similar fatal complications in the future (Gilbey et al., 2012). Cases of death during or following PDT in which the technique is related to the cause of death have only been reported in a small number of cases. Almost all fatal complications of PDT result from vascular injury (Gilbey et al., 2012). Any vascular pulsation palpated over the tracheostomy site mandates preoperative ultrasound or conversion to open surgical tracheostomy. Patients with previous neck surgery, radiotherapy or unclear surgical anatomy should be regarded with caution. If a difficult intubation or a difficult procedure is anticipated, it may be preferable not to attempt PDT with a plan to convert to surgical tracheostomy if necessary but instead to perform surgical tracheostomy without attempting PDT. This preliminary study sought to determine the success of photodynamic therapy (PDT) in reducing lesion size in an effort to assess the potential application of this treatment approach in a neoadjuvant role. Objectives. To quantify the effects of PDT on lesion area mm2 for basal cell and squamous cell carcinomas of the face (Jeremic et al., 2011). Eighteen participants (10 BCC lesions and 8 SCC lesions of the face) were assessed. Four lesions (all from the BCC group) showed a complete response to PDT. PDT as a neoadjuvant treatment may provide a simple, efficient, and viable approach to reducing the area of malignant lesions of the face with the advantage of reduced cosmetic and aesthetic morbidities. Photodynamic therapy and photothermal therapy (PTT) using nanoparticles have gained significant attention for its therapeutic effect for cancer treatment. In the present study, fabricated polypyrrole nanoparticles by employing bovine serum albumin-phycocyanin complex and the formulated particles were stable in various physiological solutions like water, phosphate buffered saline and culture media. The formulated nanoparticles did not cause any noticeable toxicity to MDA-MB-231 and HEK-293 cells (Bharathiraja et al., 2018). The obtained nanoparticles effectively killed MDA-MB-231 cells in a dual way upon laser illumination, one is through phycocyanin propagated reactive oxygen species upon laser illumination and in another way it eradicated the treated cells by converting optical energy into heat energy. Additionally, the nanoparticles generated good amplitude of ultrasound signals under photoacoustic imaging (PAT) system that facilitates imaging of treated cells. In conclusion, the fabricated particles could be used as a multimodal therapeutic agent for treatment of cancer in the biomedical field (Bharathiraja et al., 2018). The objective of the present study was to analyse the currently available methods and possibilities for antimicrobial photodynamic therapy in medicine with special reference to otorhinolaryngology. The results of the treatment of 300 patients with various suppurative ENT pathologies using antimicrobial PDT were subjected to the analysis (Lapchenko et al., 2014). It made it possible to elucidate the mechanisms and parameters of photodynamic treatment and to reveal disadvantages of the modern methods of antimicrobial photodynamic therapy. Special attention is given to the management of acute inflammation in the laryngopharynx and to the topical problems of up-to-date antimicrobial PDT (Lapchenko et al., 2014). Photodynamic therapy is an exciting area of current research. As discussed in this chapter, some successful clinical applications of this entity have been developed. Selective use of photodynamic therapy currently is of benefit to highly selected patients and holds the potential of help with some problems not currently well treated. The potential utility of photodynamic therapy coupled with other cancer therapies is very intriguing. The whole area of photodynamic therapy in viral disease is just being opened to clinical investigation. As laser technology improves and as laboratory experience with known photosensitizers continues and new photosensitizers are developed, more significant clinical contributions will surely be made (Davis, 1990). Alternative treatments are needed to achieve consistent and more complete port wine stain (PWS) removal, especially in darker skin types; photodynamic therapy is a promising alternative treatment. It is essential to understand treatment tissue effects to design a protocol that will achieve selective vascular injury without ulceration and scarring. The objective of this work is to assess skin changes associated with TS-mediated PDT with clinically relevant treatment parameters (Moy et al., 2017; (Moy et al., 2017). TS-mediated PDT at 0.75 mg/kg combined with 15 and 25 J/cm2 light doses resulted in vascular injury with minimal epidermal damage. At light dose of 50 J/cm2, epidermal damage was noted with vascular injury (Moy et al., 2017). At light doses >50 J/cm2, both vascular and surrounding tissue injury were observed in the forms of vasculitis, extravasated red blood cells, and coagulative necrosis. Extensive coagulative necrosis involving deeper adnexal structures was observed for 75 and 100 J/cm2 light doses. Observed depth of injury increased with increasing radiant exposure, although this relationship was not linear (Moy et al., 2017). TS-mediated PDT can cause selective vascular injury; however, at higher light doses, significant extra-vascular injury was observed. This information can be used to contribute to design of safe protocols to be used for treatment of cutaneous vascular lesions. Photodynamic therapy represents a palliative treatment resulting in induction of inflammatory reactions with importance for the development of an antitumor immunity (Zecha et al., 2016; Strand et al., 2017; Krowchuk et al., 2019; Whelan. et al., 2019; Klimza et al., 2019; Jackowska et al., 2018; Mosca et al., 2019; Jain et al., 2016; Dehkordi et al., 2015; Lou et al., 2019). Cancer/testis antigens have been associated with poor prognosis in different types of cancer, including head and neck squamous cell carcinoma (Theodoraki et al., 2016). Tumor tissue samples before and after PDT were evaluated for the expression of four different CTAs by immunohistochemistry. Expression intensity and subcellular expression pattern were assessed (Theodoraki et al., 2016). To describe the outcomes of bedside percutaneous dilatational tracheostomy (PDT) extended to the care of high-risk patients in the intensive care unit (ICU) by the use of suspension laryngoscopy to secure the airway (White et al., 2010). PDT is considered untenable or when transport to the operating room for a standard open tracheostomy is considered too cumbersome or potentially dangerous (White et al., 2010). Photodynamic therapy is an established treatment modality, used mainly for anticancer therapy that relies on the interaction of photosensitizer, light and oxygen (Zecha et al., 2016; Strand et al., 2017; Krowchuk et al., 2019; Whelan. et al., 2019; Klimza et al., 2019;, 2018; Mosca et al., 2019; Jain et al., 2016; Dehkordi et al., 2015; Lou et al., 2019).

For the treatment of pathologies in certain anatomical sites, improved targeting of the photosensitizer is necessary to prevent damage to healthy tissue (Kaščáková et al., 2014). Investigation of the uptake and photodynamic activity of conjugates in-vitro in human erythroleukemic K562 cells showed that conjugation of [Tyr3]-octreotate with Ce6 in conjugate 1 enhances uptake (by a factor 2) in cells over-expressing sst2 compared to wild-type cells. Co-treatment with excess free Octreotide abrogated the phototoxicity of conjugate 1 indicative of a specific sst2-mediated effect. In contrast conjugate 2 showed no receptor-mediated effect due to its high hydrophobicity. When compared with un-conjugated Ce6, the PDT activity of conjugate 1 was lower (Liu et al., 2017). Both glucocorticoids and H1-antihistamines are widely used on patients with airway diseases. However, their direct effects on airway epithelial cells are not fully explored (Zecha et al., 2016; Strand et al., 2017; Krowchuk et al., 2019; Whelan. et al., 2019; Klimza et al., 2019; Mosca et al., 2019; Jain et al., 2016; Dehkordi et al., 2015; Lou et al., 2019).

Therefore, the primary culture of human nasal epithelial cells (HNEpC) to delineate *in vitro* mucosal responses to above two drugs. HNEpC cells were cultured with/without budesonide and azelastine. The growth rate at each group was recorded and measured as population double time. Concentration-dependent treatment-induced inhibition of HNEpC growth rate was observed. Cells incubated with azelastine proliferated significantly slower than that with budesonide and the combined use of those drugs led to significant PDT prolong (Liu et al., 2017). The objective of this study was to investigate a new technique for tracheal puncture during percutaneous dilatational tracheotomy. A new invention, known as SafeTrach, was used: this instrument allows exact localization of the puncture site with built-in protection of the posterior tracheal wall. Surgery was performed on 17 patients with this technique, and our experience is described in this report (Zecha et al., 2016; Strand et al., 2017; Krowchuk et al., 2019; Whelan. et al., 2019; Klimza et al., 2019; Mosca et al., 2019; Jain et al., 2016; Dehkordi et al., 2015; Lou et al., 2019).

The results showed that this new technique minimizes known risk factors compared with existing PDT techniques, including patients with disadvantageous anatomy (Margolin et al., 2017).

CONCLUSION

- The use of photomedicine offers a number of opportunities to improve the survival and quality of life of these patients. Although multiple rounds of PDT are often required, the side effects are much less severe than those seen with the three conventional treatments - surgery, radiation therapy, and chemotherapy

- Clinical interest in laser induced fluorescence spectroscopy (LIF) and photodynamic therapy is growing rapidly and could eventually lead to the close parallel use of these techniques. However, differences in LIF due to photosensitiser retention as well as tissue damage and healing processes can interfere with autofluorescence diagnostic methods. Therefore, residual photosensitizing fluorescence is likely to influence some LIF-based diagnostic techniques at a time when patients are at high risk of tumor recurrence.

REFERENCES

Ahn, PH; Finlay, JC; Gallagher-Colombo, SM; Quon, H; O'Malley, Jr. BW; Weinstein, GS; Chalian, A; Malloy, K; Sollecito, T; Greenberg, M; Simone, 2nd. CB; McNulty, S; Lin, A; Zhu, TC; Livolsi, V; Feldman, M; Mick, R; Cengel, KA; Busch, TM. Lesion oxygenation associates with clinical outcomes in premalignant and early stage head and neck tumors treated on a phase 1 trial of photodynamic therapy. *Photodiagnosis Photodyn Ther*, 2018, 21, 28-35.

Alexander W Eckert, Matthias HW Lautner, Andreas Schu¨tze, Helge Taubert. Johannes Schubert & Udo Bilkenroth. Coexpression of hypoxia-inducible factor-1a and glucose transporter-1 is associated with poor prognosis in oral squamous cell carcinoma patients. *Histopathology*, 2011, 58, 1136–1147.

Alexander W Eckert, Matthias HW Lautner, Andreas Schu¨tze, Helge Taubert. Johannes Schubert & Udo Bilkenroth. Coexpression of hypoxia-inducible factor-1a and glucose transporter-1 is associated with poor prognosis in oral squamous cell carcinoma patients. *Histopathology*, 2011, 58, 1136–1147.

Al-Qahtani, K; Adamis, J; Tse, J; Harris, J; Islam, T; Seikaly, H. Ultra percutaneous dilation tracheotomy vs mini open tracheotomy. A comparison of tracheal damage in fresh cadaver specimens. *BMC Res Notes*, 2015, 8, 237.

Argiris, A; Karamouzis, MV; Raben, D; Ferris, RL. Head and neck cancer. *Lancet.*, 2008, 371(9625), 1695-709.

Atkins, Jr. JP; Keane, WM; Young, KA; Rowe, LD. Value of panendoscopy in determination of second primary cancer. A study of 451 cases of head and neck cancer. *Arch Otolaryngol*, 1984, 110(8), 533-4.

Augustin, R. The Protein Family of Glucose Transport Facilitators: It's Not Only About Glucose After All. *IUBMB Life*, 2010, 62(5), 315–333.

Barasch, MR; Migliorati, A; Milstein, CA; Genot, DM; Lansaat, MT; van der Brink, LR; Muhanna, N; Chan, HHL; Townson, JL; Jin, CS; Ding, L; Valic, MS; Douglas, CM; MacLaughlin, CM; Chen, J; Zheng, G; Irish, JC. Photodynamic therapy enables tumor-specific ablation in preclinical models of thyroid cancer. *Endocr Relat Cancer*, 2020 Feb, 27(2), 41-53.

Bharathiraja, S; Manivasagan, P; Moorthy, MS; Bui, NQ; Jang, B; Vy Phan, TT; Jung, WK; Kim, YM; Lee, K. D; Oh, J. Photo-based PDT/PTT dual model killing and imaging of cancer cells using phycocyanin-polypyrrole nanoparticles. *Eur J Pharm Biopharm*, 2018, 123, 20-30.

Biesaga, B. Regulacja ekspresji białka HIF 1 jako nowa strategia celowanej terapii nowotworów złośliwych [Regulation of HIF 1 protein expression as a new strategy for targeted cancer therapy]. NOWOTWORY *Journal of Oncology* 2008, 58(3), 255–259.

Boppana, NB; Stochaj, U; Kodiha, M; Bielawska, A; Bielawski, J; Pierce, JS; Korbelik, M; Separovic, D. C6-pyridinium ceramide sensitizes SCC17B human head and neck squamous cell carcinoma cells to photodynamic therapy. *J Photochem Photobiol B*, 2015, 143, 163-8.

Cancer. 2016 Jun, 24(6), 2793-805. doi: 10.1007/s00520-016-3153-y. Epub 2016 Mar.

Cerrati, EW; Nguyen, SA; Farrar, JD; Lentsch, EJ. The efficacy of photodynamic therapy in the treatment of oral squamous cell carcinoma: a meta-analysis. *Ear Nose Throat J.*, 2015, 94(2), 72-9.

Chatterjee, S; Rhee, Y; Chung, PS; Ge, RF; Ahn, JC. Sulforaphene Enhances The Efficacy of Photodynamic Therapy In Anaplastic

Thyroid Cancer Through Ras/RAF/MEK/ERK Pathway Suppression. *J Photochem Photobiol B*, 2018, 179, 46-53.

Chen, WH; Lecarosb, RLG; Tsengc, YC; Huangc, L; Hsud, YC. Nanoparticle delivery of HIF1α siRNA combined with photodynamic therapy as a potential treatment strategy for head-and-neck cancer, *CancerLett.*, 2015, 359(1), 65-74.

Chen-Xi Li, Jia-Lin Sun, Zhong-Cheng Gong, Zhao-Quan Lin, Hui Liu. Prognostic value of GLUT-1 expression in oral squamous cell carcinoma A prisma-compliant meta-analysis. *Medicine*, (2016), 95, 45.

Civantos, FJ; Karakullukcu, B; Biel, M; Silver, CE; Rinaldo, A; Saba, NF; Takes, RP; Vander Poorten, V; Ferlito, A. A Review of Photodynamic Therapy for Neoplasms of the Head and Neck. *Adv Ther.*, 2018, 35(3), 324-340.

Cohen, O; Shnipper, R; Yosef, L; Stavi, D; Shapira-Galitz, Y; Hain, M; Lahav, Y; Shoffel-Havakuk, H; Halperin, D; Adi, N. Bedside percutaneous dilatational tracheostomy in patients outside the ICU: a single-center experience. *J Crit Care*, 2018, 47, 127-132.

Davis, RK. Photodynamic therapy in otolaryngology-head and neck surgery. *Otolaryngol Clin North Am*, 1990, 23(1), 107-19.

de Bruijn, HS; Brooks, S; van der Ploeg, A; van den Heuvel; Ten Hagen, TLM; de Haas, ERM; Robinson, DJ. Light Fractionation Significantly Increases the Efficacy of Photodynamic Therapy Using BF-200 ALA in Normal Mouse Skin. *PLoS One*, 2016, 11(2), e0148850.

Dehkordi, MA; Einolghozati, S; Ghasemi, SM; Abolbashari, S; Meshkat, M; Behzad, H. Effect of low-level laser therapy in the treatment of cochlear tinnitus: a double-blind, placebo-controlled study. *Ear Nose Throat J.*, 2015 Jan, 94(1), 32-6.

Denise Hélen Imaculada Pereira de Oliveira 1, Ericka Janine Dantas da Silveira, Ana Miryam Costa de Medeiros, Pollianna Muniz Alves, Lélia Maria Guedes Queiroz. Study of the etiopathogenesis and differential diagnosis of oral vascular lesions by immunoexpression of GLUT-1 and HIF-1α. *J Oral Pathol Med*, 2014, 43(1), 76-80.

Even-Tov, E; Koifman, I; Rozentsvaig, V; Livshits, L; Gilbey, P. Pre-procedural Ultrasonography for Tracheostomy in Critically Ill Patients: A Prospective Study. *Isr Med Assoc J*, 2017, 19(6), 337-340.

Fang, X; Wu, P; Li, J; Qi, L; Tang, Y; Jiang, W; Zhao, S. Combination of apoptin with photodynamic therapy induces nasopharyngeal carcinoma cell death *in vitro* and *in vivo*. *Oncol Rep*, 2012, 28(6), 2077-82.

Furuta, Y; Tsushima, N; Nakazono, A; Fukuda, A; Kimura, S; Takahashi, H; Tsubuku, T; Matsumura, M. [Introduction of Percutaneous Dilational Tracheotomy in Otolaryngology Residency Training]. *Nihon Jibiinkoka Gakkai Kaiho*, 2015, 118(12), 1443-8.

Gadkaree, SK; Schwartz, D; Gerold, K; Kim, Y. Use of Bronchoscopy in Percutaneous Dilational Tracheostomy, *JAMA Otolaryngol Head Neck Surg*, 2016, 142(2), 143-9.

Gilbey, P. Fatal complications of percutaneous dilatational tracheostomy. *Am J Otolaryngol*, 2012, 33(6), 770-3.

Gronkiewicz, Z; Krzeski, A; Kukwa, W. Wybrane markery biologiczne w niektórych zmianach naczyniowych głowy i szyi. Selected biological markers in various vascular lesions of the head and neck. *Postepy Hig Med Dosw*, 2014, 68, 1206-1215.

Hang Yang, Jiang-Tao Zhong, Shui-Hong Zhouand, He-Ming Han. Roles of GLUT-1 and HK-II expression in the biological behawior of head and neck cancer. *Oncotarget*, 2019, Vol. 10, (No. 32), pp. 3066-3083.

He, C; Liu, D; Lin, W. Self-assembled core-shell nanoparticles for combined chemotherapy and photodynamic therapy of resistant head and neck cancers. *ACS Nano*, 2015; 9(1):991-100.

Sterenborg, HJCM; Ten Hagen, TLM; Robinson, DJ; van Hagen, MP. Somatostatin analogues for receptor targeted photodynamic therapy. *PLoS One*, 2014, 9(8), e104448.

Jain, A; Frampton, SJ; Sachidananda, R; Jain, PK. *Use of potassium titanyl*, Jan, 143(1), e20183475. doi: 10.1542/peds.2018-3475. PMID: 30584062.

Jeremic, G; Brandt, MG; Jordan, K; Doyle, PC; Yu, E; Moore, CC. Using photodynamic therapy as a neoadjuvant treatment in the surgical excision of nonmelanotic skin cancers: prospective study. *J Otolaryngol Head Neck Surg*, 2011, 40 Suppl 1, S82-9.

Jeremic, G; Moore, CC; Brandt, MG; Doyle, PC. Neoadjuvant use of photodynamic therapy in Basal cell and squamous cell carcinomas of the face. *ISRN Dermatol*, 2011, 2011, 809409.

Johnson-Obaseki, S; Veljkovic, A; Javidnia, H. Complication rates of open surgical versus percutaneous tracheostomy in critically ill patients. *Laryngoscope.*, 2016, 126(11), 2459-2467.

Justin E Swartz 1, Ajit J Pothen 1, Inge Stegeman 1 2, Stefan M Willems 3, Wilko Grolman. Clinical implications of hypoxia biomarker expression in head and neck squamous cell carcinoma: a systematic review. *Cancer Med*, 2015, 4(7), 1101-16.

Justin E. Swartz, Ajit J. Pothen, Inge Stegeman1,2, Stefan M. Willems3 & Wilko Grolman. Clinical implications of hypoxia biomarker expression in head and neck squamous cell carcinoma: a systematic review. *Cancer Medicine*, 2015, 4(7), 1101–1116.

Kaščáková, S; Hofland, LJ; De Bruijn, HS; Ye, Y; Achilefu, S; van der Wansem, K; van der Ploeg-van den Heuvel, A; van Koetsveld, PM; Brugts, MP; van der Lelij, A.

Kehinde Adekolaa, b; Steven T. Rosena, b; and Mala Shanmugam. Glucose transporters in cancer metabolism. *Curr Opin Oncol.*, 2012, 24(6), 650–654.

Kehinde Adekolaa, b, Steven T. Rosena, b, Mala Shanmugam. Glucose transporters in cancer metabolism. *Curr Opin Oncol.*, 2012, 24(6), 650–654.

Khalid Al-Qahtani 1 2, Jon Adamis 3, Jennifer Tse 4, Jeffery Harris 5, Tahera Islam 6, Hadi Seikaly. Ultra percutaneous dilation tracheotomy vs mini open tracheotomy. A comparison of tracheal damage in fresh cadaver specimens. *BMC Res Notes*, 2015, 8, 237.

Kim, H; Kim, SW; Seok, KH; Hwang, CW; Ahn, JC; Jin, JO; Kang, HW. Hypericin-assisted photodynamic therapy against anaplastic thyroid cancer. *Photodiagnosis Photodyn Ther.*, 2018, 24, 15-21.

Lapchenko, AS. [Photodynamic therapy. The fields of applications and prospects for the further development in otorhinolaryngology]. *Vestn Otorinolaringol*, 2015, 80(6), 4-9.

Lapchenko, AS; Gurov, AV; Kucherov, AG; Order, RI; Ioannides, GF. [Modern approaches to antimicrobial and anti-inflammatory photodynamic therapy in otorhinolaryngology]. *Vestn Otorinolaringol*, 2014, (1), 60-3.

Lee, SJ; Hwang, HJ; Shin, JI; Ahn, JC; Chung, PS. Enhancement of cytotoxic effect on human head and neck cancer cells by combination of photodynamic therapy and sulforaphane. *Gen Physiol Biophys*, 2015, 34(1), 13-21.

Liu, SC; Lin, CS; Chen, SG; Chu, YH; Lee, FP; Lu, HH; Wang, HW. Effect of budesonide and azelastine on histamine signaling regulation in human nasal epithelial cells. *Eur Arch Otorhinolaryngol*, 2017, 274(2), 845-853.

Buckmiller, LM; Richter, GT; Suen, JY. Diagnosis and management of hemangiomas and vascular malformations of the head and neck. *Oral Diseases*, (2010), 16, 405–418.

Lu, K; He, C; Lin, W. Nanoscale Metal–Organic Framework for Highly Effective Photodynamic Therapy of Resistant Head and Neck Cancer. *J Am Chem Soc.*, 2014, 9(1), 991-1003.

Lou, Z; Gong, T; Kang, J; Xue, C; Ulmschneider, C; Jiang, JJ. The Effects of Photobiomodulation on Vocal Fold Wound Healing: *In Vivo* and *In Vitro* Studies. *Photobiomodul Photomed Laser Surg.*, 2019 Sep, 37(9), 532-538.

Macheda, M; Rogers, S; Best, J. Molecular and Cellular Regulation of Glucose Transporter (GLUT) Proteins in Cancer. *J Cell Physiol*, 202, 654–662, (2005).

Mallidi, S; Khan, AP; Liu, H; Daly, L; Rudd, G; Leon, P; Khan, S; Hussain, BMA; Hasan, SA; Siddique, SA; Akhtar, K; August, M; Troulis, M; Cuckov, F; Celli, JP; Hasan, T. Platform for ergonomic intraoral photodynamic therapy using low-cost, modular 3D-printed components: Design, comfort and clinical evaluation. *Sci Rep*, 2019, 9(1), 15830.

Manivasagan, P; Bharathiraja, S; Moorthy, M. S; Mondal, S; Seo, H; Lee, KD; Oh, J. Marine natural pigments as potential sources for therapeutic applications. *Crit Rev Biotechnol*, 2018, 38(5), 745-761.

Marchal, S; Dolivet, G; Lassalle, HP; Guillemin, F; Bezdetnaya, L. Targeted photodynamic therapy in head and neck squamous cell carcinoma: heading into the future. *Lasers in Medical Science*, 2015, 30(9), 2381-2387.

Margolin, G; Ullman, J; Karling, J. A New Technique for Percutaneous Tracheotomy. *Otolaryngol Head Neck Surg*, 2017, 156(5), 966-968.

Marius G. Bredell1, Jutta Ernst1, Ilhem El-Kochairi1, Yuliya Dahlem1, Kristian Ikenberg, Desiree M. Schumann. Current relevance of hypoxia in head and neck cancer. *Oncotarget*, 2016, 7(31), 50781-50804.

Marius G. Bredell1, Jutta Ernst1, Ilhem El-Kochairi1, Yuliya Dahlem1, Kristian Ikenberg, Desiree M. Schumann. Current relevance of hypoxia in head and neck cancer. *Oncotarget*, 2016, 7(31), 50781-50804.

Moy, WJ; Yao, J; de Feraudy, SM; White, SM; Salvador, J; Kelly, KM; Choi, B. Histologic changes associated with talaporfin sodium-mediated photodynamic therapy in rat skin. *Lasers Surg Med*, 2017, 49(8), 767-772.

Nowak, A; Kern, P; Koscielny, S; Usichenko, TI; Hahnenkamp, K; Jungehülsing, M; Tittel, M; Oeken, J; Klemm, E. Feasibility and safety of dilatational tracheotomy using the rigid endoscope: a multicenter study. *BMC Anesthesiol.*, 2017 Jan 14, 17(1), 7.

Peng, W; de Bruijn, HS; Ten Hagen, TLM; Berg, K; Roodenburg, JLN; van Dam, GM; Witjes, MJH; Robinson, DJ. In-Vivo Optical Monitoring of the Efficacy of Epidermal Growth Factor Receptor Targeted Photodynamic Therapy: The Effect of Fluence Rate. *Cancers (Basel)*, 2020, 12(1), 190.

Sharwani, A; Alharbi, FA. Monitoring of photobleaching in photodynamic therapy using fluorescence spectroscopy. *Gulf J Oncolog*, 2014, 1(16), 79-83.

Song, X; Liu, X; Chi, W i wsp. Hypoxia-induced resistance to cisplatin and doxorubicin in non-small cell lung cancer is inhibited by silencing of HIF-1α gene. *Cancer Chemother Pharmacol*, 2006, 58, 776-84.

Song, X; Liu, X; Chi, W i wsp. Hypoxia-induced resistance to cisplatin and doxorubicin in non-small cell lung cancer is inhibited by silencing of HIF-1α gene. *Cancer Chemother Pharmacol*, 2006, 58, 776-84.

Suel y Nonogaki; Heloisa GA. Campos, Ossa mu Butugan, Fernando A. Soares 2, Flávia Regina Rotea Mangone 4, Humberto Torloni 2; Mit zi BrentaniRENTANI, M. Markers of vascular differentiation, proliferation and tissue remodeling in juvenile nasopharyngeal angiofibromas. *Experimental and Therapeutic MemEdicine*, 1, 921-926, 2010.

Suel y Nonoga ki1; Heloisa GA; Campos, Ossa mu Butugan 3, Fernando A. Soares 2, Flávia Regina Rotea Mangone 4, Humberto Torloni 2 and M. Mit zi BrentaniRENTANI. Markers of vascular differentiation, proliferation and tissue remodeling in juvenile nasopharyngeal angiofibromas. *Experimental and Therapeutic MemEdicine*, 1, 921-926, 2010.

Theodoraki, MN; Lorenz, KJ; Schneider, J; Thierauf, JC; Spagnoli, G; Schuler, PJ; Hoffmann, TK; Laban, S. Influence of Photodynamic Therapy on the Expression of Cancer/Testis Antigens in Squamous Cell Carcinoma of the Head and Neck. *Anticancer Res*, 2016, 36(8), 3973-82.

Theodoraki, MN; Lorenz, K; Lotfi, R; Fürst, D; Tsamadou, C; Jaekle, S; Mytilineos, J; Brunner, C; Theodorakis, J; Hoffmann, TK; Laban, S; Schuler, PJ. Influence of photodynamic therapy on peripheral immune cell populations and cytokine concentrations in head and neck cancer. *Photodiagnosis Photodyn Ther*, 2017, 19, 194-201.

Theodoraki, MN; Yerneni, SS; Brunner, C; Theodorakis, J; Hoffmann, TK; Whiteside, TL. Plasma-derived Exosomes Reverse Epithelial-to-Mesenchymal Transition after Photodynamic Therapy of Patients with Head and Neck Cancer. *Oncoscience.*, 2018, 5(3-4), 75-87.

Tsunoi, Y; Araki, K; Ozeki, E; Hara, I; Shiotani, A; Terakawa, M; Sato, S. Photoacoustic diagnosis of pharmacokinetics and vascular shutdown effects in photodynamic treatment with indocyanine green-lactosome for a subcutaneous tumor in mice. *Photodiagnosis Photodyn Ther.*, 2019, 26, 436-441.

van Leeuwen-van Zaane, F; de Bruijn, HS; van der Ploeg-van den Heuvel, A; Sterenborg, HJMC; Robinson, DJ. The effect of fluence rate on the acute response of vessel diameter and red blood cell velocity during topical 5-aminolevulinic acid photodynamic therapy. *Photodiagnosis Photodyn Ther*, 2014, 11(2), 71-81.

van Straten, D; Mashayekhi, V; de Bruijn, HS; Oliveira, S; Robinson, DJ. Oncologic Photodynamic Therapy: Basic Principles, Current Clinical Status and Future Directions. *Cancers* (Basel)., 2017, 9(2), 19.

Volgger, V; Betz, CS. Photodynamic therapy in the upper aerodigestive tract. Overview and outlook. *J Biophotonics.*, 2016, 9(11-12), 1302-1313.

Wang, CP; Lou, PJ; Lo, FY; Shieh, MJ. Meta-tetrahydroxyphenyl chlorine mediated photodynamic therapy inhibits the migration and invasion of a nasopharyngeal carcinoma KJ-1 cell line. *J Formos Med Assoc*, 2014, 113(3), 173-8.

Wei Lin, Chen-Yi Yin, Qi Yu, Shui-Hong Zhou, Liang Chai, Jun Fan, Wen-Dong Wang. Expression of glucose transporter-1, hypoxia inducible factor-1α and beclin-1 in head and neck cancer and their implication. *Int J Clin Exp Pathol*, 2018, 11(7), 3708-3717.

Wei Lin, Chen-Yi Yin, Qi Yu, Shui-Hong Zhou, Liang Chai, Jun Fan, Wen-Dong Wang. Expression of glucose transporter-1, hypoxia inducible factor-1α and beclin-1 in head and neck cancer and their implication. *Int J Clin Exp Pathol*, 2018, 11(7), 3708-3717.

Wei, MF; Chen, MW; Chen, KC; Lou, PJ; Lin, SYF; Hung, SC; Hsiao, M; Yao, CJ; Shieh, MJ. Autophagy promotes resistance to photodynamic therapy-induced apoptosis selectively in colorectal cancer stem-like cells. *Autophagy*, 2014, 10(7), 1179-92.

Weihe Zhang, a; Yi Liu, bc; Xiaozhuo Chen, bcde; Stephen, C. Bergmeier. Novel inhibitors of basal glucose transport as potential anticancer agents. *Bioorganic & Medicinal Chemistry Letters*, 20, (2010), 2191–2194.

Weihe Zhang, a; Yi Liu, bc; Xiaozhuo Chen, bcde; Stephen, C. Bergmeier. Novel inhibitors of basal glucose transport as potential anticancer agents. *Bioorganic & Medicinal Chemistry Letters*, 20, (2010), 2191–2194.

White, HN; Sharp, DB; Castellanos, PF. Suspension laryngoscopy-assisted percutaneous dilatational tracheostomy in high-risk patients. *Laryngoscope*, 2010, 120(12), 2423-9.

Wojdas, W; Kosek, J; Dżaman, K; Szczygielski, K; Ratajczak, J; Jurkiewicz, D. Zastosowanie laserów w leczeniu chorób krtani. Application of lasers in treatment of larynx diseases. *Otolaryngol Pol*, 2009, 63 (7), 76-79.

Wu, CN; Duan, SF; Mu, XT; Wang, Y; Lan, PY; Wang, XL; Li, KC. Assessment of optic nerve and optic tract alterations in patients with orbital space-occupying lesions using probabilistic diffusion tractography. *Int J Ophthalmol*, 2019, 12(8), 1304-1310.

Wuttipong Tirakotai, Sandra Fremann, Niels Soerensen, Wolfgang Roggendorf, Adrian M. Siegel, Hans Dieter Mennel, Yuan Zhu, Helmut Bertalanffy, Ulrich Sure. Biological activity of paediatric cerebral cavernomas: an immunohistochemical study of 28 patients. *Childs Nerv Syst*, (2006), 22, 685–691.

Wuttipong Tirakotai, Sandra Fremann, Niels Soerensen, Wolfgang Roggendorf, Adrian M. Siegel, Hans Dieter Mennel, Yuan Zhu, Helmut Bertalanffy, Ulrich Sure. Biological activity of paediatric cerebral cavernomas: an immunohistochemical study of 28 patients. *Childs Nerv Syst*, (2006), 22, 685–691.

Xue, K; Wang, YN; Zhao, X; Zhang, HX; Yu, D; Jin, CS. Synergistic effect of meta-tetra(hydroxyphenyl)chlorin-based photodynamic therapy followed by cisplatin on malignant Hep-2 cells. *Onco Targets Ther*, 2019, 12, 5525-5536.

Yang, S; Zhou, C; Sun, B; Wang, F; Han, Z; Zhang, H; Han, J; Shen, Y, Zhang, J. Efficacy of microsurgery in combined with topical- PDT in treating recurrent respiratory papillomatosis: compare JORRP with AORRP. *Acta Otolaryngol.*, 2019, 139(12), 1133-1139.

Zecha, JA; Raber-Durlacher, JE; Nair, RG; Epstein, JB; Elad, S; Hamblin, MR; Zecha, JA; Raber-Durlacher, JE; Nair, RG; Epstein, JB; Sonis, ST; Elad, S; Hamblin. Zhang, C; Gong, T; Wang, J; Chou, A; Jiang, JJ. Topical Application of 5-Aminolevulinic Acid Is Sufficient for Photodynamic Therapy on Vocal Folds. *Laryngoscope*, 2019, 129(2), E80-E86.

Zhang, H; Shen, B; Swinarska, JT; Li, W; Xiao, K; He, P. 9-Hydroxypheophorbide α-mediated photodynamic therapy induces matrix metalloproteinase-2 (MMP-2) and MMP-9 down-regulation in Hep-2 cells via ROS-mediated suppression of the ERK pathway. *Photodiagnosis Photodyn Ther*, 2014, 11(1), 55-62.

Zhang, QZ; Zhao, KQ; Wu, Y; Li, XH; Yang, C; Guo, LM; Liu, CH; Qu, D; Zheng, CQ. 5-aminolevulinic acid-mediated photodynamic therapy and its strain-dependent combined effect with antibiotics on Staphylococcus aureus biofilm. *PLoS One*, 2017, 12(3), e0174627.

Zhou, JC; Zhang, JJ; Zhang, W; Ke, ZY; Ma, LG; Liu, M. Expression of GLUT-1 in nasopharyngeal carcinoma and its clinical significance. *European Review for Medical and Pharmacological Sciences.*, 2017, 21, 4891-4895.

Zhou, JC; Zhang, JJ; Zhang, W; Ke, ZY; Ma, LG; Liu, M. Expression of GLUT-1 in nasopharyngeal carcinoma and its clinical significance. *European Review for Medical and Pharmacological Sciences.*, 2017, 21, 4891-4895.

ABOUT THE EDITORS

Dorota Bartusik-Aebisher
Professor
Medical College of The University of Rzeszow, Poland

Professor Dorota Bartusik-Aebisher is working at The University of Rzeszow in Poland. Professor Dorota Bartusik-Aebisher research is focused on applications of MRI to cancer treatments. Her research interests are the applications of 19F MR to drug tracking and visualization of cancer tissue. She published more than 300 scientific papers and books chapters in MRI field.

David Aebisher
Professor
Medical College of The University of Rzeszow, Poland

Professor David Aebisher is working at The University of Rzeszow in Poland. Professor David Aebisher research is focused on advancement of photodynamic therapy for clinical medicine including the development of devices for localized release of 1O2 to cancerous tissue, and overcoming the limited tissue depth to which current photodynamic therapy can be applied. He published more than 300 scientific papers and books chapters in PDT field.

INDEX

#

5- aminolevulinic acid (5-ALA), 81, 89, 108, 117
5-aminolevulinic acid (5-ALA), viii, 81, 89, 99, 101, 102, 104, 107, 117, 136, 138

A

alcohol, 3, 76
anti-cancer therapy, viii, 113

B

biochemical studies, vii
biochemistry, 1

C

cancer, v, vii, viii, 1, 13, 14, 16, 17, 18, 19, 20, 21, 22, 23, 24, 25, 27, 32, 33, 34, 35, 36, 37, 38, 39, 40, 41, 42, 43, 44, 45, 46, 47, 48, 49, 51, 52, 53, 54, 55, 57, 61, 62, 63, 64, 65, 66, 69, 70, 71, 72, 77, 78, 79, 80, 81, 82, 89, 94, 97, 99, 100, 101, 103, 104, 105, 106, 107, 108, 109, 110, 111, 112, 113, 115, 129, 130, 132, 133, 135, 136
cancer assessment, viii, 51
cancer risk, viii, 13, 27, 33
carcinogens, viii, 27
cases, viii, 1, 4, 12, 20, 31, 35, 41, 62, 69, 87, 94, 97, 102, 114, 129
chemotherapy, vii, 2, 12, 13, 18, 20, 21, 22, 28, 36, 48, 55, 58, 62, 63, 65, 71, 72, 78, 79, 82, 98, 114, 127, 131
CT, 15, 16, 17, 18, 24, 32, 38, 70
cytotoxic reactive oxygen species, vii, viii, 81, 88, 113, 115

D

disease, 2, 13, 19, 26, 28, 49, 52, 54, 55, 58, 71, 72, 86, 91, 99, 104, 116
DNA, 2, 21, 39, 52, 100
dysphagia, viii, 27, 85, 96, 101

E

environment, viii, 27

H

head, v, vii, viii, 1, 2, 10, 11, 12, 13, 14, 15, 16, 17, 18, 19, 20, 21, 22, 23, 24, 25, 26, 28, 33, 34, 35, 36, 37, 39, 40, 41, 42, 43, 44, 45, 46, 47, 48, 51, 52, 53, 54, 57, 61, 62, 63, 64, 65, 66, 67, 69, 70, 71, 72, 77, 78, 79, 80, 81, 82, 89, 94, 95, 98, 99, 100, 101, 102, 103, 104, 105, 106, 107, 108, 109, 110, 112, 113, 114, 128, 129, 130, 131, 132, 133, 134, 135, 136
head and neck cancer, vii, 2, 11, 12, 13, 14, 15, 16, 17, 18, 19, 20, 21, 22, 23, 24, 26, 28, 33, 34, 36, 37, 44, 48, 52, 53, 54, 57, 62, 63, 64, 65, 66, 67, 69, 71, 72, 77, 78, 79, 80, 83, 90, 99, 103, 106, 109, 110, 112, 114, 129, 131, 133, 134, 135, 136
head and neck cancer biomarkers, vii
head and neck cancer treatments, vii
head cancer(s), vii, 1, 2, 11, 51
histological appearance, viii, 51

I

interactions, vii, viii, 46, 52, 81
investigation, viii, 34, 81, 84, 116, 126

L

laryngeal cancer, 21, 27, 28, 32, 52, 100, 105, 121
larynx, viii, 1, 4, 19, 28, 32, 52, 53, 55, 58, 63, 67, 69, 73, 79, 94, 108, 114, 137
light, vi, vii, viii, 81, 82, 91, 94, 97, 99, 105, 110, 111, 113, 114, 130
lower pharynx, viii, 1
lymph nodes, viii, 2, 51, 53, 57
lymph nodes status, viii, 51

M

malignancy, viii, 18, 51, 56, 74
markers, 34, 37, 39, 44, 52, 53, 55, 69, 70, 71, 72, 78, 79, 80, 92, 106, 121, 131, 135
medications, viii, 81
metabolic state, viii, 32, 69
metastases, viii, 7, 15, 16, 30, 51, 55, 57, 70, 73
molecular diagnostics, viii, 3, 51
morbidity, viii, 51, 59, 72, 83, 116
mortality, viii, 19, 51, 72, 94, 115
mouth, viii, 1, 2, 11, 52, 95, 114
MRI, 2, 12, 18, 20, 32, 52, 59, 70

N

neck, v, vii, viii, 1, 2, 10, 11, 12, 13, 14, 15, 16, 17, 18, 19, 20, 21, 22, 23, 24, 25, 26, 27, 32, 33, 35, 36, 37, 39, 41, 42, 43, 45, 46, 47, 51, 52, 53, 54, 55, 57, 61, 62, 63, 64, 65, 66, 69, 70, 71, 72, 77, 78, 79, 80, 81, 82, 89, 94, 95, 98, 99, 100, 101, 102, 103, 104, 105, 106, 107, 108, 109, 113, 114, 128, 129, 130, 131, 132, 133, 134, 135
neck cancer, vii, viii, 2, 14, 20, 27, 32, 51, 52, 53, 55, 57, 63, 72, 85, 91, 96, 114, 130
neoplastic cells, viii, 51, 86, 115
normal tissue, vii, viii, 6, 56, 57, 81, 91, 98, 117

O

oxygen, viii, 82, 97, 113, 115

P

palliative major surgery, vii, 113
palliative treatment, vii, 87, 89, 116
patients, vii, 1, 2, 11, 12, 13, 14, 16, 17, 18, 19, 20, 21, 22, 25, 26, 28, 33, 36, 37, 38, 40, 42, 44, 45, 47, 52, 54, 55, 57, 61, 63, 64, 65, 72, 79, 82, 89, 94, 98, 102, 103, 109, 114, 127, 128, 130, 131, 132, 135, 137
PDT, vii, viii, 81, 82, 89, 94, 98, 100, 102, 103, 104, 107, 108, 109, 113, 126, 127, 129, 137
pharynx, 10, 55, 73, 114
phenomenon, vii, viii, 9, 29, 81
photodynamic diagnosis (PDD), vii, viii, 81
Photodynamic therapy, vii, viii, 81, 94, 113
photodynamic therapy (PDT), vii, viii, 62, 63, 64, 65, 81, 82, 89, 94, 97, 98, 99, 100, 101, 102, 103, 104, 105, 106, 107, 108, 109, 110, 111, 112, 113, 126, 127, 128, 129, 130, 131, 132, 133, 134, 135, 136, 137, 138
photosensitizer emitting fluorescence, vii, viii, 81
photosensitizers, vii, viii, 81, 82, 90, 94, 97, 98, 99, 101, 114
photosensitizing agent (PS), viii, 64, 84, 97, 100, 105, 113, 129, 133

R

radiology, viii, 3, 51, 52
reactive oxygen, vii, viii, 81, 88, 113, 115
reactive oxygen species, 82, 115
response, viii, 2, 35, 40, 42, 47, 51, 55, 58, 61, 73, 79, 86, 89, 95, 98, 103, 108, 116, 136

S

significant problem, vii, 1, 4
smoking, viii, 10, 27, 76
squamous cell, vii, viii, 1, 4, 15, 16, 18, 19, 20, 21, 26, 27, 32, 33, 36, 38, 43, 48, 51, 54, 57, 58, 62, 63, 65, 71, 72, 78, 82, 89, 95, 97, 100, 102, 105, 106, 108, 109, 111, 113, 116, 128, 129, 130, 132, 134
squamous cell carcinoma, vii, viii, 1, 4, 15, 16, 18, 19, 20, 21, 26, 27, 32, 33, 36, 38, 43, 48, 51, 52, 54, 57, 58, 62, 63, 65, 71, 72, 78, 82, 89, 95, 97, 100, 102, 105, 106, 108, 109, 111, 113, 116, 128, 129, 130, 132, 134
status, 33, 34, 110, 112, 136
stridor, viii, 27
symptom, viii, 2, 27

T

targeted therapies, viii, 69
therapy, vii, viii, 2, 12, 16, 17, 18, 21, 28, 34, 37, 42, 43, 47, 54, 58, 61, 62, 63, 64, 65, 67, 72, 77, 78, 79, 80, 81, 82, 89, 94, 97, 98, 99, 100, 101, 102, 103, 104, 105, 107, 108, 109, 110, 111, 112, 113, 127, 129, 130, 133, 134, 135, 136, 138
throat, viii, 1, 2, 11, 24, 114, 129, 130
toxicity, 13, 56, 59, 72, 91, 115
traditional diagnostic methods, viii, 51
treatment toxicity, viii, 60, 69
treatment(s), v, vii, viii, 1, 12, 14, 15, 17, 18, 19, 20, 22, 23, 24, 26, 28, 35, 36, 44, 51, 52, 54, 57, 62, 63, 64, 66, 67, 69, 70, 71, 72, 77, 78, 79, 82, 89, 94, 97, 100, 101, 104, 106, 107, 108, 109, 111, 112, 114, 126, 127, 129, 130, 131, 136, 137
tumor eradication, viii, 88, 113
tumor grading, viii, 51

tumor(s), vii, viii, 1, 2, 12, 13, 14, 17, 20, 21, 22, 24, 28, 33, 35, 36, 37, 38, 39, 40, 41, 43, 44, 45, 46, 47, 48, 51, 52, 53, 54, 55, 57, 58, 61, 62, 63, 64, 66, 69, 70, 71, 72, 78, 79, 80, 81, 82, 89, 94, 97, 98, 99, 103, 105, 106, 110, 111, 113, 114, 128, 129, 136

V

voice alteration, viii, 27

W

women, viii, 27, 59